A Consumer Guide to

INTERPRETING YOUR BLOOD WORK

HOW TO READ IT AND NATURAL WAYS TO IMPROVE YOUR RESULTS

Dr. Daniel T. Wagner

Interpreting Your Blood Work: How to Read It and Natural Ways to Improve Your Results
© 2016
Dr. Daniel T. Wagner

All rights reserved. Reproduction or translation of any part of this book through any means without permission of the copyright owner is unlawful, except for promotional use. Request for other permissions or further information should be addressed in writing to the author. This book is not intended as a substitute for professional medical advice. The reader should consult the appropriate healthcare professional regarding specific needs.

ISBN-13: 978-1532722066
ISBN-10: 1532722060

Editor: Gina Mazza
Cover Design and Interior Layout: Lee Ann Fortunato-Heltzel,
Creative One Marketing

Dr. Daniel T. Wagner
Wildwood, PA
Askdrdanwagner@gmail.com

DEDICATION

To my mother . . .

You've inspired me with love, humility, honesty and a genuine work ethic.

TABLE OF CONTENTS

Introduction i

Who Needs to Get a Blood Test? 1

How to Interpret the Data in This Book:
    Understanding the Numbers 5

The Blood Tests 7
    Acid Phosphatase 7
    Adenosine Triphosphate (ATP) 8
    Adrenal Function 9
    Alanine Transaminase (ALT) (SGPT) 9
    Albumin 10
    Albumin/globulin ratio 11
    Aldolase 11
    Aldosterone 12
    Alkaline Phosphate 12
    Alpha Fetoprotein AFP 13
    Ammonia 14
    Amylase 14
    Angiotensin Converting Enzyme (ACE) 15
    Anion Gap 15
    Antibody Tests, serum 16
    Antinuclear Antibody (ANA) 16
    Antithrombin III 17
    Apolipoprotein (Apo B) 18
    Aspartate Aminotransferrase (AST)(SGOT) 18
    Basophils, Absolute 19
    Bilirubin 20
    Bilirubin, Direct 21
    Blood Gases, Arterial (ABG) 21
    Blood Group (Type A,O,B,AB) 22
    Blood Urea Nitrogen (BUN) 23

BUN/Creatinine Ratio 24
Body Mass Index (BMI) 25
Calcium, serum 25
Cancer Antigen CA-125..26
Cancer Antigen CA-15-3 27
Candida Albicans Antibodies 28
Carbon Dioxide (CO2)..29
Carbon Monoxide (CO) 30
Carcinoembryonic Antigen (CEA) 30
Cardio C-reactive Protein (CRP)...31
Catecholamines 32
CD-57 (Lyme disease)...32
Chloride 33
Cholesterol, total serum 34
Chlolesterol/HDL Ratio..35
Coagulation Factors 36
Complete Metabolic Panel (CMP) 36
Copper, serum...36
Cortisol 37
Creatinine 38
Creatinine Phosphokinase 39
Cyclic Citrulline PEP IgG (CCP) 40
DHEA 41
eGFR 42
Electrolytes 43
Eosinophils, Abs..43
Estradiol 44
Estriol 45
Estrone..46
Ferritin..47
Fibrinogen 48
Folic Acid 49
Follicle Stimulating Hormone (FSH) 49
Free Thyroxine Index (FTI) 50
Galactose Transferase (GALT) 51
Gamma Globulins (see Immunoglobulins)...................................51
Gamma Glutamyl Transferase 52

TABLE OF CONTENTS

Gastrin 52
Glomerular Filtration Rate (GFR) 53
Glucocorticoids 54
Glucose 54
Glucose Fasting 55
Glutathione, serum 55
Glycohemoglobin (GHb) 56
Granulocytes 56
Haptoglobin 57
HDL Cholesterol 58
Hematocrit 58
Hemoglobin HgB 59
Hemoglobin A1C 60
HLA B-27 Antigen 60
Homocysteine 61
Human Chlorionic Gonatropin 62
Human Growth Hormone 62
Human Papillomavirus 63
Immunoglobulins 64
IgA 65
IgE 66
IgG 66
IgM 67
International Normalization Ratio (INR) 68
Insulin, serum 69
Insulin-like Growth Hormone (IGF-1) 70
Iodine, serum 70
Iron, serum (Fe) 72
Iron-binding Capacity (TIBC) 73
Lactic Acid 73
Lacto Dehyrogenase (LDH) 74
LDL Cholesterol 75
Lead, serum 76
Lipase 77
Liver, serum 78
Lipoprotein-associated Phospholipase (Lp-PLA2) 79
Lyme Disease (see CD-57) 80

Lymphocytes, Abs 81
Magnesium, serum 82
Manganese, serum 83
Mean Cell Hemoglobin (MCH) 84
Mean Cell Hemoglobin Conc. (MCHC) 85
Mean Corpuscular Hemoglobin (MCV) 85
Mercury, serum 86
Monocytes, Abs. 87
Myelocytes % 88
Myeloproxidase (MSA) 88
Myoglobin 89
Neutrophils, Abs 90
5' Nucleotidase 91
Osmolality 91
Oxygen Saturation (SO2) 92
Parathyroid 92
Partial Pressure of Carbon Dioxide (PCO2) 93
Partial Thrombin Time (PCO2) 94
pH 94
Phenylalanine 96
Phosphorus, serum 96
Platelets (Thrombocytes) 97
Porphobilinogen (PBG) 98
Porphyrins 99
Potassium, serum 100
Pregnenolone, serum (P5) 101
Progesterone, serum 102
Prolactin 104
Prostate Specific Antigen (PSA) 104
Protein, total 105
Prothrombin Time (PT) 106
Red Blood Cells (RBCs) 107
Red Cell Distribution (RDW) 108
Renin 108
Resin T3 Uptake 109
Retic Count 109
Reticulocytes 109

TABLE OF CONTENTS

Rheumatoid Factor (RF) 110
Sedimentation Rate (ESR) 111
Serotonin 112
Sex Hormone Binding Globulin (SHBG) 113
Sodium 113
Sodium Bicarbonate 114
Testosterone, serum 115
Thyroglobulin Antibodies 117
Thyroid Peroxidase Antibodies (TPO) 117
Thyroid Stimulating Hormone (TSH) 118
Thyroid Symptoms (Hypothyroid) 119
Thyroid Symptoms (Hyperthyroid) 120
Thyroxine Binding Globulin (TBG) 121
Thyroxine, serum (T4) 121
Thyroxine, T4 Free 122
TORCH 123
Total Iron-binding Globulin (TIBC) 123
Transferrin Saturation (TSAT) 124
Triiodothyronine, serum (T3) 124
T3, Free (FT3) 124
T3, Reverse (rT3) 125
Triglycerides 125
Troponin I 126
Uric Acid 127
Viral Hepatitis 128
Vitamin A, serum 129
Vitamin B12, serum 129
Vitamin C, serum 130
Vitamin D, serum 131
VLDL 132
White Blood Cells (WBCs) 133
White Blood Cell Differential 134
Zinc, serum 135

Appendix 137
    Adrenal Function Tests 137
    Antibody Serum Tests..138
    Cardiac Function Tests 138
    Complete Metabolic Blood Panel (CMP) 139
    DHEA Normal Serum Levels 139
    Estrogen Dominance...140
    Kidney Renal Function Tests 140
    Liver/Gall Bladder Individual Function Tests 141
    Pathogen Serum Test 141
    Pregnancy Serum Tests 142
    pH Values 142
    Thyroid Function Tests...143
    Cancer Serum Tests 143

Measurements 145

Index 147

About the Author 151

INTRODUCTION

"It all looks Greek to me."

This is a typical response that my patients have regarding the report that accompanies the blood work results that they get from their physician. As an integrative health practitioner, my patients often share with me that they've obtained blood work from their medical doctor but no one took the time to explain what the results meant. Their doctor saying, "everything looks good" doesn't quite suffice, especially for those who want to truly be in charge of their own health. What do the high and low numbers indicate? Are they good or bad? Are they average or in the danger zone?

After more than 18 years of practicing integrative medicine, I've come to believe that blood screening tests are extremely valuable, and the results of these screenings should be something that anyone with a body should understand. Blood chemistry is a very effective tool that any healthcare practitioner can use to screen and identify imbalances in body functions and metabolism. Fortunately for patients, blood laboratory tests are relatively inexpensive and, in most cases, are covered by medical insurances.

A comprehensive blood chemistry panel will allow your physician to have quick access to understanding your degree of health or disease. It also enables the practitioner to establish a baseline of biomarkers that can be used to track "outcomes" over time to determine if the conventional and/or alternative medical professionals on your healthcare team (in either a treatment or an advisory/consultative role) are making progress.

In my private practice, I use blood chemistry as a crucial marker to evaluate how the implementation of energy "frequency" medicine is working in combination with my recommendations of diet, nutrition, homeopathy, vitamins, herbs, amino acids, exercise and stress-management techniques. Some scientists and physicians have called frequency medicine the "medicine of the future." It is based on our knowledge of quantum mechanics and the effects it has on a biological system. Every organ and cell in the human body has its own distinct wave frequency, or oscillation (much like every cell phone has its own frequency as a phone number). These frequencies—which represent the exchange of information between a particular tissue or cell and the environment—can now be measured.

I wrote Interpreting *Your Blood Work* for you, the average consumer, to help you to decipher your blood test results and use this knowledge to your health advantage. The language and format have been simplified so that you can more easily grasp the often confusing medical terminology and "jargon", and perhaps better understand why your physician or integrative practitioner may have ordered the test in the first place. (I have made every effort to include the most current data possible.) The information in this book is NOT meant for self-diagnosis or self-treatment (leave that to the professionals!) nor is it meant to replace your doctor. It can, however, better inform you about the state of your health and greatly improve your dialogue with your healthcare team. Use it as a valuable tool and resource, not as an ultimate authority.

What gives *Interpreting Your Blood Work* a different twist from other books that define common blood tests is that I include natural alternatives to traditional medications that I have researched first hand in my practice. There are myriad ways to approach decisions about your health condition(s), and the addition of nutritional supplements should never be ruled out. I have seen evidence that natural interventions may improve outcomes over time. I have no interest in getting my patients to discontinue their drug therapy or decrease dosages on their own. This is never advisable; however, an increasing number of people are interested in more natural approaches to improving their overall health. Medical professionals may or may not approve of alternative approaches but nonetheless, I am dedicated to helping patients make the most informed decisions they can when responding to any health afflictions that may be uncovered via blood chemistry testing. Of course, I encourage you to openly discuss with your healthcare professional everything you take or practice outside of orthodox medicine (drugs, surgery and psychotherapy).

Above all, keep in mind that you have a right to this information! It is your blood work. So, I encourage you to ask for a copy of your results the next time these tests are ordered by your doctor. Do not hesitate to ask questions about them. Even if your blood results are normal, it is a good practice to discuss them with your doctor (or at least a physician's assistant, nurse or nurse practitioner). I realize that most physicians today are pressed for time—statistics show that a patient in the US has just nine minutes on average with his or her physician during a visit—but it is your prerogative as their patient to ask them to *make* the time to talk with you.

It is my sincere wish and intent that this book helps you to make better and more informed choices with regard to your health. Remember, you are behind the wheel of the car of life, and only you can make decisions on which way to turn and what your final destination will be. Ultimately, the decision is yours as to what efforts you choose to make to improve your overall health, vitality and well-being.

Many blessings to you in both body and spirit!
Dr. Dan

Who Needs to Get a Blood Test?

Generally, the answer to the above question is "just about everyone", but unless you ask, you might not find out what your blood test results really mean for your health. I've said it once already yet it bears repeating: Spending the time to unravel the mystery of your test results is well worth the effort, since your blood panel can reveal quite a bit of information that is quite indicative of your overall health status.

What are some of the typical routine blood tests?

Routine tests include a complete blood count (CBC) to measure your white and red blood cell numbers, platelets, hemoglobin, hematocrit and other numbers. This test can uncover anemia, oxygen levels, infections from bacteria and/or virus, and even cancer in the blood.

Another common blood test is the basic metabolic panel. It checks for kidney and liver function, heart health, glucose, minerals and electrolyte levels. This is usually associated with a lipoprotein panel that measures high-density cholesterol (HDL), the good cholesterol, bad cholesterol (LDL), triglycerides and other fats in your blood.

Looking for signs of inflammation is a major reason to get blood work done. The process by which inflamed arteries lead to cardiovascular disease, including heart attack and stroke, is generally invisible except for a tracer test called a C-reactive protein (CRP).

All women (and men to a lesser degree) can benefit from getting a thyroid panel. Symptoms of an underactive thyroid (hypothyroidism) have many common symptoms such as weight gain, hair loss, dry skin, foggy memory and sleep disturbances. With an overactive thyroid (hyperthyroidism) there may be signs of a goiter (a swollen area in the neck), increased heart rate, anxiety, weight loss and loose stools.

Since more than 200,000 American men are diagnosed with prostate cancer each year, tracking their prostate-specific antigen (PSA) can flag early problems. Although not an exact science, high levels can be an early sign of carcinoma, but likewise can be a benign enlargement or a bacterial infection known as prostatitis.

As you can surmise, blood tests are invaluable in helping physicians check for certain diseases and conditions. They also help to check the function of your organs and show how well treatments and/or drug therapies are working. The following tests should be considered just about every time you have a complete physical: CBC, kidney and liver panel, lipid (cardiac) panel, blood glucose, and a periodic vitamin D level.

What Your Doctor May Not Always Tell You About Your Results

Again, ask your doctor to discuss all of your blood tests results with you. Frequently, patients assume that "no news is good news." Even if your doctor says there is nothing of concern in your results, do not take this as a final analysis. If your blood glucose, cholesterol and other blood chemistry fall within normal ranges, this is excellent and it means that the doctor's office may not reach out to you about your report.

Even if things appear normal, insist on discussing your results with your health practitioner for the following reasons.

- What is considered "normal" may differ between men and women. If you compare your blood results with someone else's, you may be surprised to find differences. A woman's results can even vary during menstruation, or pre- versus post-menopause.

- Results can also differ depending on your age. Children generally have much lower "normal" levels of hemoglobin than adults. Most "normals" for cholesterol, HDL and LDL are based on a 27-year-old male or female. People age 60 and older obviously do not have the body of a 27-year-old, so their normal will naturally be different.

- False-negative and false-positive tests happen. I alert my patients about these occasional "kinks" in the system because accuracy is critical and meaningful when dealing with your health. An example is the rapid HIV test, for which false positives are common. Other viruses, including Hepatitis C come back negative, but the infection can be present and not realized. Fungal infections are also well known to produce false results.

- Test values can differ from lab to lab. In my research, I've found this to be the most disconcerting fact of all. Each lab may have a different reference range on what is considered "normal." This fact is even recognized by the US Food and Drug Administration, so don't be surprised if you find that a prior blood test report varies from hospital to hospital, or from older to newer tests.

- Abnormal results are not necessarily due to a disease state. Yes, an abnormal test could lead to a disease or disorder; however, outcomes can also be abnormal for many other reasons. The time of the day when the blood is drawn may be a factor. The time of fasting before the procedure may also precipitate inaccurate results. Taking certain medications or natural products before the test can skew results, as can recent recovery from a cold, flu or virus.

- Mistakes can happen! Although mix-ups of patients' blood samples are rare, they do happen by accident or by technician stress and overwork. How your blood sample is handled even before it is analyzed can affect results, too.

In general, keep in mind that a "positive" result may not always be positive, and likewise a "negative" result does not always mean bad news. Repeating blood tests after receiving untoward results is not unreasonable; in fact, it may be wise and advisable.

Your doctor most likely cannot and will not diagnose many diseases and medical problems with blood tests alone. Other factors include external signs and symptoms, your medical history, your vital signs (like blood pressure, pulse and temperature) and results from other tests such as a urinalysis, saliva and/or stool testing. As I see in my practice all the time, extracurricular issues not generally investigated by the conventional medical community may have repeatedly untoward effects on your blood results. These include things like heavy metal toxicity, radiation, e-smog, pesticides, herbicides, food additives, genetically modified foods and other environmental chemicals.

How to Interpret the Data in This Book:

Understanding the Numbers

For your convenience, I have alphabetically listed the blood tests to show whether the levels of different substances in your body fall within normal range. For many blood tests, the normal range is the range seen in 95 percent of healthy people in a certain group. For other tests, normal ranges vary depending on age, gender, race, disease state(s) and other factors.

Generally, your blood results may fall outside the normal range for many reasons. Other factors such as diet, medications (both prescription and other-the-counter), dietary supplements, physician activity or inactivity, alcohol or marijuana use and abuse, and menstrual cycles can also cause abnormal results.

Your doctor has to determine if abnormal results might be a sign of disease or disorders and, ideally, should discuss any abnormal or unusual tests with you or a designated family member. As stated earlier, however, this discussion time does not always happen due to busy schedules, time constraints, and ongoing restrictions by insurance companies and managed-care companies that unfortunately trickle down from practitioner to patient. Perhaps one way of looking at the content of this book is to "know before you go." Having accurate information about the irregularities of your blood work the next time you get a blood test can empower you to ask the right questions to your doctor.

To use this book, first refer to the tests in the Blood Tests section of the book. Each blood test listing gives information on the highs and lows beyond the "normal" levels established by the medical community. It also suggests natural ways to improve your results (be it dietary, vitamin supplements, herbal, homeopathic or essential oils), and includes extra notes on additional information pertinent to the specific test. At the end of the blood test listings, you will find an appendix to better categorize a number of tests that pertain to a medical condition. This is done for your easy reference.

The Blood Tests

Acid Phosphatase (AP) (1.0-1.9 IuL)

A category of enzymes produced mainly in the bones and liver, alkaline phosphatase enzymes are responsible for splitting off the acidic mineral phosphorus, creating an alkaline balance. High blood levels of alkaline phosphatase could be indicative of bone or liver disease. In the case of children or adolescents, high levels may simply reflect rapid bone growth. If your blood test reveals high levels, you will need to discuss potential underlying conditions with your physician.

The acid phosphatase enzyme is primarily in the male prostate that, in effect, is a male PAP test (blood and the prostate gland). AP is a family of enzymes found widely in nature (plants and animals). Mystery surrounds its precise functional role.

- HIGH: anemia, blood clots, bone disease, cancer, diabetes, heart attack, hepatitis, kidney disease, overactive parathyroid, pneumonia, prostate disorder

- FALSE HIGH: clofibrate, androgen hormones, stimulation of prostate exam

- LOW: not significant, alcohol use

- FALSE LOW: fluoride

- Ways to improve your results (to lower): Fish and milk (sources of vitamin D), higher copper foods (cashews), sardines, herring, cod liver oil, Shiitake mushrooms.

- Ways to improve your results (to keep from increasing): In contrast, foods rich in zinc should be avoided since zinc is an important structured component of the metalloprotein. These zinc-rich foods include tuna, beef liver, lamb, shellfish, corn oil, cheese, coconut oil and carbonated beverages.

- Helpful nutrients (to lower): extra vitamin D2 and D3 supplements

Adenosine Triphosphate (ATP)

ATP is an energy-bearing molecule found in all living cells. Formation of nucleic acids, transmission of nerve impulses, muscle contraction and many other energy-consuming reactions of metabolism are made possible by the energy in ATP molecules. The energy in ATP is obtained from the breakdown of foods.

- LOW (Hypophosphatemia): certain blood cancers such as lymphoma or leukemia, hereditary causes, liver failure, ketoacidosis, osteomalacia, hyperparathyroidism, chronic fatigue syndrome, mitochondrial diseases

- FALSE LOW: low serum levels of calcium and phosphorus

- Ways to improve your results: Alkalize the blood (e.g., minerals, lemons, limes, chlorella, spirulina, sodium bicarbonate) and exercise.

- Helpful nutrients: milk thistle, vitamin C, B-complex vitamins

- Note: Check patient's oxygen level. See a qualified practitioner for advice.

Adrenal Function

The adrenal glands are part of the endocrine system (located on the top of the kidneys). The adrenal cortex produces aldosterone hormone, sex hormones (estrogen and androgens) and cortisol. They regulate the levels of sodium in the body, which increases energy, responds to stress(ors) and helps regulate blood pressure. There are three types of adrenal hormones:

- GLUCOCORTICOIDS influence protein and carbohydrate metabolism. They regulate the production of sugar from protein to rise when blood sugars fall.

- MINERALCORTCOIDS influence sodium and potassium levels

- ANDROGENS influence secondary male characteristics including testosterone levels

- See Adrenal Function Tests in the Appendix.

Alanine aminotransaminase (ALT), formally known as serum glutamic-pyruvic transaminase (SGPT) (10-34 IU/L)

ALT is an enzyme produced primarily in the liver, skeletal and heart muscle. Often ordered in conjunction with AST, ALT is a test to detect liver damage. ALT increases in the instance of liver disease, but may also rise from injuries, tumors or drug reactions.

- HIGH: liver cell damage, heart failure, infection, bile duct failure, cirrhosis, liver tumor, jaundice, burns, severe shock, muscle trauma, pancreatitis

- FALSE HIGH: antibiotics, antidepressants, alcohol, NSAIDs, beta blockers, cortisone, narcotics, birth control pills

- LOW: desirable; however, look for malnutrition

- Ways to improve your results: Improve your diet by eating organic fruits and vegetables. Coffee can help and less consumption of alcohol. Add more fiber.

- Helpful herbs: milk thistle (silymarin)
- See Antibody Serum Test in the Appendix.

Albumin, serum (3.9-5.0 g/dL)

A primary blood protein produced in the liver by Human Growth Hormone (HGH) and made from the protein foods we eat every day. Albumin is the main constituent (largest portion, 60%) of total blood protein. Albumin is a fluid part of the blood and keeps the water content of blood over 90%. Albumin maintains how thick or thin the blood is (directly affecting blood pressure).

- HIGH: almost always a dehydration problem, leaking blood vessels, excess protein in the urine (kidney damage), possible vitamin A deficiency, Wilson's disease
- FALSE HIGH: high protein diet, burns
- LOW: chronic liver disease (cirrhosis, hepatitis, ascites), blood protein disorders, kidney disease, low thyroid, inability to fight infections, after weight-loss surgery, Crohn's disease, burns, low protein diet
- FALSE LOW: anticoagulant drugs, protein deficiency, burns, diarrhea, pregnancy
- Ways to improve your results: Egg whites are good food sources. Drink more water and alkalize the body's pH.
- Helpful nutrients: Boost immunity with supplements such as CoQ10, vitamin C, resveratrol, vitamin D3, omega-3 fatty acids
- See Complete Metabolic Blood Panel, Kidney Renal Function Tests, Liver/Gall Bladder Individual Function Tests and Pregnancy Serum Tests in the Appendix.

Albumin/Globulin Ratio (1.0-2.5%)

A/G ratio is an alternative way to tell if albumin or globulin levels in the blood are abnormal. It is used to evaluate different liver and kidney diseases, as well as check the nutritional status of the patient.

- HIGH: rare, lack of water. May be caused by high production of immunoglobulins (e.g., IgM, IgG, IgA that can lead to allergies). May be seen in hypothyroidism and leukemia
- LOW: may indicate overproduction of globulins (proteins in the blood) in conditions such as multiple myeloma, inflammation, syphilis, RA, liver disease, and some autoimmune diseases, burns
- Ways to improve your results: Lower the inflammatory response by creating an alkalize pH, hydrate with more water, adding minerals, add lemons or limes to water. Take 1 level teaspoon on sodium bicarbonate.
- Helpful nutrients: Omega-3 fatty acids, extra vitamin C (to lower histamine levels)
- Helpful herbs: curcumin, boswellia

Aldolase, serum (1.0-7.5 U/ml)

Aldolase is a protein (called an enzyme) that helps break down certain sugars to produce energy. It is found in high amount in muscle tissue.

- HIGH: heart attack, skeletal muscle disease or damage, lead poisoning, stoke, hepatitis, viral infections (MONO), liver damage, pancreatic or prostate cancer
- LOW: not important
- Ways to improve your results: Follow recommendations used to lower cholesterol levels.

Aldosterone, serum (1-9 ng/dl)

The aldosterone blood test measures the level of the hormone aldosterone in blood. Aldosterone is a hormone released by the adrenal glands. It helps the body regulate blood pressure. Aldosterone increases the reabsorption of sodium and water and the release of potassium in the kidneys. This action raises blood pressure.

- HIGH: kidney disease, cancer (adrenal tumor), liver disease, a very low sodium diet

- LOW: adrenal gland disease (Addison's), diabetes, very high sodium diet

- Ways to improve your results: Support the adrenal glands with stress management. Eat more fruits and vegetables. Use basil, rosemary, essential oils.

- Helpful nutrients: B-complex, vitamin B5, vitamin C, Co-enzyme Q10, L-tyrosine, raw adrenal cortex, magnesium, potent multi-vitamin

- Helpful herbs: astragalus, chlorophyll, shiitake mushrooms, shiitake mushrooms, Siberian ginseng

- See Adrenal Function Tests in Appendix.

Alkaline Phosphatase (ALP) (44-147 IU/L)

Alkaline phosphatase is an enzyme in the cells lining the biliary ducts of the liver, bones, kidneys and intestines. ALP is also present placental tissue, so it is higher in growing children and after bone fractures.

- HIGH: bile duct obstruction, cancer, high cholesterol levels, over-active parathyroid disease, gall stones, diseases of the liver, diabetes, hepatitis, bone tumors, elderly with Pageant's disease (bone diseases), Lyme disease

- LOW: may be seen with blood transfusions, kidney disease, scurvy, malnutrition, underactive parathyroid disease, heart bypass surgery, magnesium, zinc deficiencies

- Ways to improve your results: Low ALP by eating more foods rich or fortified with vitamin D (e.g., fish, nonfat dairy products, shitake mushrooms). Eat healthy fats (e.g., coconut oil, nuts, seeds, olive oil, avocados.

- Helpful nutrients (to raise ALP): Supplement with more zinc if levels are low. Eat more foods high in zinc (e.g., beef, pork, shellfish, cheese, lentils, coconut oil, carbonated beverages). Add phosphorus, vitamin A, vitamin B12

- Helpful nutrients (to lower ALP): Add vitamin D (if deficient). Scrutinize Rx drug regimen. Avoid foods high in zinc.

- See Complete Metabolic Blood Panel, Liver/Gall Bladder Individual Function Tests and Pregnancy Serum Tests in Appendix.

Alpha-fetoprotein (AFP) (up to 2.5 mg/dL)

Alpha fetoprotein (AFP) is a protein produced by the liver and yolk sac of a fetus. AFP has no normal function in adults. The alpha fetoprotein test (AFP) is a blood test performed to measure, diagnose or monitor fetal distress or fetal abnormalities. It can also detect some liver disorders and some cancers (primary hepatocellular carcinoma) in adults.

- HIGH: possible defects in the developing fetus, particularly spinal cord and brain, liver cancer, germ-cell tumors, ataxia

- FALSE HIGH: twins, older fetus

- LOW: possible chromosomal problems in fetus (Down's syndrome)

- FALSE LOW: fetus is younger

- Note: AFP has a low rate of accuracy (about 60%) and has come under criticism for alarming parents.

- See Cancer Serum Tests in the Appendix

Ammonia, serum (15-45 mcg.dL)

Ammonia is a major by-product of protein breakdown in the body (mainly the intestines). The liver then converts this ammonia into urea, which is then excreted in the urine, Ammonia levels are generally measured to check the functioning of the liver in cases of extreme drowsiness and even check for cirrhosis of the liver. In liver failure, ammonia builds up in the blood.

- HIGH: excess alcohol, Reye's syndrome (in children), a high protein diet, bleeding in stomach, liver disease, heart failure, parasitic invasion

- LOW: not important

- Ways to improve your results: Set up an effective detoxification regimen with a qualified practitioner.

- Helpful nutrients: lemons, grapefruit seeds, arginine, ornithine

Amylase, serum (28-100 IU/L)

Amylase is a digestive enzyme (from the pancreas and salivary glands) that digests carbohydrates (starches) or polysaccharides into smaller disaccharide units. The enzyme eventually converts them into monosaccharides such as glucose. People who can't digest fats often eat sugar and carbohydrates to make up for the lack of fat in their diet. If their diet is excessive in carbohydrates, they develop an amylase deficiency.

- HIGH: acute pancreatitis, alcoholism, cystic fibrosis

- LOW: liver disease, Parkinson's disease, mercury or lead poisoning

- FALSE LOW: stimulants, glaucoma meds

- Ways to improve your results (for low levels): Supplement with a multi-digestive enzyme containing protease, amylase, cellulose, lactase and a phosphorus deficiency.

- Note: Take 5 to 15 minutes before larger meals for improved absorption. Check with a qualified practitioner.

Angiotensin Converting Enzyme (ACE) (9-67 U/L)

The ACE test measures the level of angiotensin-converting enzyme (ACE) in the blood. This test is commonly ordered to help diagnose and monitor a disorder called sarcoidosis. People with sarcoidosis may have their ACE level tested regularly to check how severe the disease is and how well treatment is working.

- HIGH: higher than normal ACE levels may be a sign of sarcoidosis (an inflammatory lung disease) as ACE levels rises or falls as sarcoidosis worsens or improves, Hodgkin disease, diabetes, liver disease, kidney disease, COPD, multiple sclerosis, asthma

- LOW: steroid therapy, anorexia nervosa, hypothyroidism

- Ways to improve your results: See a qualified practitioner for ways to naturally treat and improve auto-immune conditions.

- Note: The use of an ACE-inhibitor anti-hypertensive drug may cause ACE levels to fall.

Anion Gap (AG) (8-16 mEq/L)

Anion Gap represents the concentration of all unmeasured anions (atoms that gain electrons) in plasma. These negatively charged proteins account for 10% of plasma anions. The acidic anions (sulfate, lactate) are produced during metabolic acidosis. The bicarbonate anions (H+) are carbon dioxide produced via the excretion from the lungs. Anion gap measures the difference between the sum of potassium and sodium ions.

- HIGH: acidosis likely due to diabetes mellitus, buildup of lactic acid, possible kidney failure in time, dehydration

- FALSE HIGH: aspirin, salicylic acid

- LOW (Hyponatremia): a decreased level of sodium in the blood, malnutrition, possible multiple myeloma (cancer of the bone marrow), excess vitamin D, hyper-parathyroidism

- FALSE LOW: lithium

- Ways to improve your results (if too high): Drink more water, eat less animal protein, and supplement with B-vitamins and extra vitamin B1 (thiamine). Alkalize your pH and take extra vitamin D.

- Ways to improve your results (if too low): Lower alkalinity, minimize intake of calcium and vitamin D, increase protein consumption.

Antibody Tests, serum

Antibodies are proteins made by the body's natural defense system (immune system) to fight foreign substances, such as bacteria. Antibodies attach themselves to the foreign substance, allowing other immune system cells to attack and destroy the substance.

The surfaces of viruses, fungi, and bacteria contain markers called antigens. To destroy these invaders, the immune system creates antibodies that are specific for each antigen.

Antinuclear Antibody (ANA) (positive/negative)

Antinuclear antibodies (ANAs, also known as antinuclear factor or ANF) are autoantibodies that bind to contents of the cell nucleus. In normal individuals, the immune system produces antibodies to foreign proteins (antigens) but not to human proteins (autoantigens).

The ANA test is a sensitive screening test used to detect autoimmune diseases. Autoimmune diseases feature a misdirected immune system, and each of them has characteristic clinical manifestations that are used to make the precise diagnosis. The interpretation or identification of a positive ANA test does not make a diagnosis. It simply suggests to the doctor to consider the possibility that an autoimmune disease is present.

Frequently, ANAs are found in patients with a number of different autoimmune diseases, such as systemic lupus, Sjögren's syndrome, rheumatoid arthritis, polymyositis, scleroderma, Hashimoto's thyroiditis, juvenile diabetes mellitus, Addison disease, vitiligo, pernicious anemia, glomerulonephritis and pulmonary fibrosis. ANAs can also be found in patients with conditions that are not considered classic autoimmune diseases, such as chronic infections and cancer.

- POSITIVE: a positive ANA test result means that autoantibodies are present. In a person with signs and symptoms, this suggests the presence of an autoimmune disease, but further evaluation is required to assist in making a final diagnosis

- NEGATIVE: ANA test must be accompanied by symptoms, since antibodies alone, with no symptoms, do not diagnose disease

- Ways to improve results: See a qualified practitioner for ways to naturally treat and improve auto-immune conditions.

- Note: If a patient has symptoms plus diagnostic antibodies or biopsy proof of disease, the patient has systemic lupus.

- See Antibody Serum Tests in the Appendix.

Antithrombin III (80-120%)

Antithrombin III (AT III) is a protein that helps control blood clotting. A blood test can determine the amount of AT III present in your body. Normal value ranges may vary slightly among different laboratories. Talk to your doctor about the meaning of your specific test results.

- HIGH: use of anabolic steroids

- LOW: increased risk of bleeding (e.g., deep vein thrombosis, phlebitis, vein inflammation, pulmonary embolus or blood clots traveling to lung)

Apo B100 (50-150 mg/dL)

The Apolipoprotein B (Apo B) test is used, along with other lipid tests, to help determine an individual's risk of developing cardiovascular disease (CVD). This test is not used as a general population screen but may be ordered if a person has a family history of heart disease and/or high cholesterol and triglycerides. It may be performed, along with other tests, to help diagnose the cause of abnormal lipid levels, especially when someone has elevated triglyceride levels.

Apo B100 is a protein that plays a role in moving cholesterol around your body. It is a form of low density lipoprotein (LDL). Mutations (changes) in apoB100 can cause a condition called familial hypercholesterolemia T. This is a form of high cholesterol that is passed down in families (inherited). It is the main protein constituent of lipoproteins such as very low-density lipoproteins (VLDL) and LDL. Concentrations of Apo B tend to mirror those of LDL-C.

- HIGH: cardiovascular disease, atherosclerosis, diabetes, elevated LDL and triglycerides, pregnancy, kidney disease

- LOW: hyperthyroidism, malnutrition, Reye syndrome, surgery, cirrhosis, severe illness

- Ways to improve your results: See HDL, Triglycerides

Aspartate aminotransferase (AST), formally known as serum glutamic-oxaloacetic transaminase (SGOT) (10-35 IU/L)

AST (SGOT) is an enzyme found in the liver and in cardiac, kidney, pancreas and skeletal muscle. AST may rise in liver and muscle disorders. AST rises 2-20 times in 4-6 hours after a heart attack, but can return to normal in 4-6 days. AST will rise 100 times when liver cells are damaged in chemical poisonings and viral hepatitis.

- HIGH: liver damage (viral or alcoholic hepatitis), heart attack, chemical poisoning, inflammation, pancreas inflammation, anemia, blood clot, Mono, pulmonary embolism, jaundice, Reye's s syndrome, pneumonia (associated with elevated HDL)

- FALSE HIGH: antibiotics, non-steroidal anti-inflammatory drugs (NSAIDs), birth control pills, blood thinners, cortisone, narcotics, gout medications

- LOW: or mid-range is ideal

- Ways to improve your results (lower SGOT): Improve your diet by eating organic fruits and vegetables, drink coffee, consume less alcohol, add more fiber, reduce fatty and high salty foods, vitamin D, B-complex and exercise.

- Helpful herb: milk thistle

- See Cardiac Function Tests, Complete Metabolic Blood Panel, Liver/Gall Bladder Individual Function Tests and Pregnancy Serum Tests in the Appendix.

Basophils, Absolute (0.0-0.2 109 cells/L) (0-200 cells/mcL) (0.5-1.0%)

Basophilic granulocytes (basophils) are the least common of the 5 white blood cells. When activated, basophils release many components (including histamine and interlukin-4) in response to an allergic (inflammatory) reaction. They are considered phagocytic. Basophils comprise only 0.01-0.03% of circulating white blood cells.

- HIGH: some leukemias (CML), rare allergic reactions (e.g. hives, food allergies), inflammation (e.g., ulcerative colitis, rheumatoid arthritis), allergic reactions (e.g., hives, food allergies), myeloma, hypothyroidism, enlarged spleen, radiation, sinusitis, Crohn's disease, Hodgkin's lymphoma, parasites, viral infections, hemolytic anemia

- LOW: not medically significant, extreme stress

- Ways to improve your results: Boost immunity and eat a whole-food diet.

- Helpful nutrients: omega-3 fatty acids, quercetin, vitamin C, N-Acetyl cysteine

- Helpful herbs: butterbur, stinging nettles, frankincense oil

- Note: (See Eosinophils)

Bilirubin, total (0.1-1.9 mg/dL)

This test measures the breakdown of heme (a part of hemoglobin in red blood cells). The liver is responsible for clearing the blood of bilirubin. Bilirubin is excreted by the liver as part of bile (enzyme stored in the gall bladder). It is helpful in evaluating liver function and evaluating jaundice (yellowing of the skin).

- HIGH: causes yellowing of skin and eyes (jaundice). This can occur in liver disease (hepatitis, cirrhosis), bile obstruction, sickle cell anemia, pernicious anemia, blood transfusions

- LOW: trauma with a large hematoma, Gilbert's disease, hemolytic anemia

- FALSE LOW: excessive use of vitamin C

- Ways to improve your results (to lower): Consume foods such as radishes, nuts, and coconut water.

- Helpful nutrients (to lower): vitamin C, selenium, B-complex, digestive enzymes, antioxidant therapy

- Helpful herbs (to lower): milk thistle, artichoke, echinacea, goldenseal, sugarcane

- See Complete Metabolic Blood Panel and Liver/Gall Bladder Individual Function Tests in the Appendix.

Bilirubin, direct (0.2-1.2 mg/dL)

Direct bilirubin is a specific form of bilirubin that is formed in the liver and excretes in the bile. Normally, very little is of this form of bilirubin is found in the blood; however, in liver disease, this form of bilirubin leaks into the blood.

- HIGH: indicates a problem with liver cells

Blood Gases, Arterial (ABG)

Blood gases are a measurement of how much oxygen and carbon dioxide are in your blood. They also determine the acidity (pH) of your blood. A blood gas analysis is ordered when someone has symptoms of an oxygen/carbon dioxide or pH imbalance, such as difficulty breathing, shortness of breath, nausea or vomiting. It may also be ordered when someone is known to have a respiratory, metabolic or kidney disease and is experiencing respiratory distress.

When someone is "on oxygen" (ventilation), blood gases may be measured at intervals to monitor the effectiveness of treatment. Other treatments for lung diseases may also be monitored with blood gases. Blood gases may also be ordered when someone has head or neck trauma, which may affect breathing. Interpreting an arterial blood gas (ABG) is a crucial skill for physicians, nurses, respiratory therapists, and other health care personnel. ABG interpretation is especially important in critically ill patients. Normal values will vary from lab to lab. They are also dependent on elevation above sea level as a person's blood oxygen level will be lower if they live higher than sea level.

Measurements include partial pressure of oxygen (PaO2), arterial pressure of carbon dioxide (PaCO2), arterial blood pH, oxygen saturation (SaO2), bicarbonate (HCO3). If left untreated, these conditions can create an imbalance that can eventually become life-threatening. A health practitioner can provide the necessary medical intervention to regain normal acid/base balance, but the underlying cause of the imbalance must also be addressed.

pH result	Bicarbonate result	PaCO$_2$ result	Condition	Common causes
< than 7.35	Low	Low	Metabolic acidosis	Kidney failure, shock, diabetic ketoacidosis, intoxication with methanol, salicylate, ethanol
> than 7.45	High	High	Metabolic alkalosis	Chronic vomiting, low blood potassium, heart failure, cirrhosis
< than 7.35	High	High	Respiratory acidosis	Narcotics, lung disease such as asthma, COPD, airway obstruction
>than 7.45	Low	Low	Respiratory alkalosis	Hyperventilation, pain, anxiety, brain trauma, pneumonia, certain drugs (e.g., salicylate, catecholamines)

Blood Groups (A, B, O, AB)

This blood grouping is also referred to as "blood typing." Blood is primarily identified (grouped) in four categories as to what proteins are on the surface of the red blood cell.

- Type A
- Type B
- Type AB found in only 2.5% of population
- Type O

Nutrients recommended per blood type:

- Type A: vitamin B12, folate, vitamin C, vitamin E, zinc, iron (only if low), calcium, selenium, quercetin, digestive enzymes
- Type B: magnesium
- Type AB: vitamin C, selenium, zinc
- Type O: B-complex, B12, folate, vitamin K
- See Antibody Serum Tests in the Appendix.

Blood Urea Nitrogen (BUN) (women: 6-20 mg/dL) (men: 8-20 mg/dL)

BUN is the waste product in your blood that comes from the breakdown of protein from the foods we eat. BUN test is the primary blood test, along with creatinine, to evaluate kidney and liver function in a wide range of circumstances.

- HIGH: suggests kidney malfunction (acute or chronic), heart failure, shock, prostate hypertrophy, dehydration, acute MI, bleeding (gastrointestinal), starvation
- FALSE HIGH: from drugs use (e.g., furosemide, methotrexate, cephalosporins, rifampin, tetracyclines, thiazide diuretics, vancomycin, spironolactone), high protein diet
- LOW: liver disease or liver failure, urinary obstruction, malnutrition, low protein diet
- How to improve your results (to lower): It is important to drink more water, lower animal protein intake, eat a more vegetarian diet, manage stress, lower blood pressure.
- Helpful nutrients (for liver integrity): L-carnitine, alpha-lipoic acid, vitamin D3, B-complex, glutathione, tyrosine
- Helpful herbs (for liver integrity): milk thistle, uva ursi, pomegranate juice, astragalus, ginkgo biloba

- See Complete Metabolic Blood Panel, Kidney Renal Function Tests and Liver/Gall Bladder Individual Function Tests in the Appendix.

BUN/Creatinine Ratio (10:1-20:1) (Older men may be a bit lower)

This test shows if your kidneys are eliminating wastes properly. The principle behind this ratio is the fact that both urea (BUN) and creatinine are freely filtered by glomerulus. Urea and creatinine are nitrogenous end products of metabolism. Urea is the primary metabolite derived from dietary protein and tissue protein turnover. Creatinine is the product of muscle creatinine catabolism.

- HIGH: if the ratio exceeds 20 it implies acute kidney injury, reduced function or possible kidney failure, increased gastrointestinal bleeding, multiple sclerosis, pancreatic insufficiency

- FALSE HIGH: steroids, prednisone

- LOW: not common, little concern, may be seen in pregnancy and malnutrition

- Ways to improve your results (to lower ratio): Drink plenty of water and stay hydrated. Eat a low protein diet. Strive for a balanced pH.

- Helpful herbs (to lower ratio): milk thistle may improve ratio, other herbs are associated with lower creatinine and blood urea nitrogen levels (e.g., nettles, chamomile, Chinese herb yin yang huo, cinnamon, Siberian ginseng, dandelion root, salvia, frankincense, myrrh, geranium, helichrysum)

- See Complete Metabolic Blood Panel, Kidney Renal Function Tests and Liver/Gall Bladder Individual Function Tests in the Appendix.

Body Mass Index (BMI) (18.5-24.9)

Body mass index (BMI) is an indication of body size—and, by association, body fat. It is calculated by multiplying your weight in pounds by 703, then dividing by height (in inches squared).

- Ways to improve your results: Follow dietary recommendations for weight loss or weight gain as needed. Check for food allergies.

- Note: To maintain weight loss, calculate how many calories you need daily by multiplying weight by 10, then add 30% to that amount.

- Helpful nutrients: conjugated linoleic acid (CLA), gamma-linolenic acid (GLA), DHEA, HGH, chitosan

- Helpful herbs: ginkgo, bladderwrack, grape seed extract, gymnema sylvestre, grapefruit essential oil

Calcium, Serum (8.5-10.4 mg/dL) (may be lower in elderly)

Calcium (Ca+) is a dominant mineral in our body. In blood, we are checking the amount of calcium not stored in bones (approximately 1 to 2%). Calcium builds bone, teeth, makes muscles work, aids in heart functions and minimizes blood clotting. Be sure to monitor the parathyroid gland (a gland next to the thyroid gland) that secretes a hormone that regulates calcium levels in our body.

- HIGH: ossification of bone, fatigue, constipation, overactive parathyroid or thyroid gland, cancer of lungs, leukemia, lymphoma, Paget's disease, associated with an increased risk of atherosclerosis, heart attack, alkalosis, bone marrow tumors, kidney problems, respiratory diseases, Celiac disease

- FALSE HIGH: excess vitamin D, antacids

- LOW: osteoporosis, osteopenia, bone disorders, underactive parathyroid, dietary deficiency (high protein), digestive issues

- FALSE LOW: pregnancy, low dairy consumption

- Ways to improve your results (to boost low levels): Supplement with calcium (citrate or hydroxyapatite) with equal amounts of magnesium and adequate vitamin D3.

- Ways to improve your results (to lower high levels): Minimize intake of dairy products and severely limit extra calcium supplementation.

- Helpful nutrients: foods high in calcium include kale, Swiss and cheddar cheese, collard greens, turnips, almonds, Brazil nuts, watercress, goat's milk and tofu

- See Complete Metabolic Blood Panel, Estrogen Dominance, Kidney Renal Function Tests and Pregnancy Serum Tests in the Appendix.

Cancer Antigen -125 (CA-125) (<35 U/ml)

CA-125 is a test used to evaluate ovarian cancer treatment. Levels above 35 U/ml are abnormal; levels above 65 consider malignant. CA-125 is a protein that is found more in ovarian cancer cells than on other cells. This protein enters the bloodstream and may be measured by a blood test.

The most common use of the test is the monitoring of women with known ovarian cancer. A decreasing level generally implies that the therapy, including chemotherapy, has been effective, while an increasing level indicates tumor recurrence. Other conditions of the ovaries and womb also produce CA-125: endometriosis, fibroids, pelvic inflammatory disease and pregnancy.

CA125 is not a completely reliable test for ovarian cancer. It shows that there is some kind of inflammation in the area of the body surrounded by hip bones (the pelvis) but it cannot tell the doctor exactly what is causing the inflammation.

- Ways to improve your results: Adjust to a more anti-cancer lifestyle and diet. Consume a more alkaline diet. Quit smoking, avoid toxins in home and workplace, exercise, minimize alcohol intake, boost immunity.

- Helpful nutrients: CoQ10, colostrum, SOD, proteolytic enzymes, vitamin C, selenium, vitamin A, flaxseed, acidophilus, multi-vitamin

- Helpful herbs: garlic, Shiitake mushrooms, frankincense and sandalwood essential oils

- See Cancer Serum Tests in the Appendix.

Cancer Antigen 15-3 (CA-15-3) (< 30U/ml)

CA 15-3 is not sensitive or specific enough to be considered useful as a tool for cancer screening. Its main use is to monitor a person's response to breast cancer treatment and to help watch for breast cancer recurrence.

CA 15-3 is sometimes ordered to give a doctor a general sense of how much cancer may be present (the tumor burden). CA 15-3 can only be used as a marker if the cancer is producing elevated amounts of it, so this test will not be useful for all people with breast cancer.

- HIGH: in general, the higher the CA 15-3 level, the more advanced the breast cancer and the larger the tumor burden

- INCREASING: increasing concentrations of CA 15-3 over time may indicate that a person is not responding to treatment or that the cancer is reoccurring

- NORMAL: normal CA 15-3 levels do not ensure that a person does not have localized or metastatic breast cancer. In some cases it may be too soon in the disease for elevated levels of CA 15-3 to be detected or the patient may be one of the 20-25% of individuals with advanced breast cancer whose tumors do not shed CA 15-3 antigens.

- MILD-MODERATE: mild to moderate elevations of CA 15-3 are seen in a variety of conditions including cancer of the lungs, pancreas, ovaries, prostate and colon, as well as non-cancerous conditions such as hepatitis, cirrhosis and benign breast disorders, akin to a certain percentage of apparently healthy individuals. The CA 15-3 elevations seen in non-cancerous conditions tend to be stable over time.

- See Cancer Serum Tests in the Appendix.

***Candida Albicans* Antibodies (<.89 EV- >1.00 EV)**

Candida is something of a controversial illness, and many medical professionals have not yet recognized it. Regretfully, this means that many patients are turned away and do not get the help that they need.

The problem is that many of the symptoms of a Candida overgrowth are quite general and can be attributed to a number of other illnesses. These days, more and more doctors are starting to diagnose candidiasis (a fungal infection typically on the skin or mucous membranes caused by *Candida albicans*.) If you can't find a qualified doctor who is willing to practice alternative medicine, try to find a local alternative practitioner who will do the tests for you.

For anti-Candida Antibodies, or the Candida Immune Complexes test, there are 3 antibodies that should be tested to measure your immune system's response to Candida: IgG, IgA, and IgM. High levels of these antibodies indicate that an overgrowth of Candida is present.
Candida antibody, IgG, IgM, IgA:
 0.89 EV or less, negative
 0.90-0.99 EV, equivocal, questionable presence
 >1.00 EV, positive, antibody detected, which may indicate current or past infection

- HIGH (POSITIVE): oral thrush, vaginal yeast infection, fungal infection on mails or skin, following chemotherapy, antibiotic use or overuse, HIV/AIDS, blood infection

- Ways to improve your results: "Starve" the Candida by starving the yeast. Eat a Candida-free diet, consume more fermented foods that help to repopulate the gut with good bacteria (e.g., kimchi, sauerkraut, kefir, yogurt and coconut water). Liver detoxification can be useful.

- Helpful nutrients: probiotics (acidophilus, saccharomyces boulardii), flaxseed, psyllium, chia seeds, caprylic acid

- Helpful herbs: oregano (wild), berberine, olive leaf, grapefruit seed extract, garlic, essential oils (e.g., melaleuca, oregano, clover, peppermint, thyme)

Carbon Dioxide (CO_2) (19-30 mmol/L)

A waste product of animal metabolism exhausted from our lungs. CO_2 starts in the body's tissues and is picked up by the blood for disposal. This test measures the dissolved CO_2 in blood. Changes in your CO_2 level may suggest that you are losing or retaining fluid. This may cause an imbalance in your body's electrolytes. CO_2 levels in the blood are affected by kidney and lung function. The kidneys help maintain the normal bicarbonate levels.

- HIGH: adrenal gland over activity, Cushing's disease, vomiting, breathing difficulties (asthma), heart disease, starvation, drug overdose, high aldosterone levels

- LOW: Addison's disease, diarrhea, alcohol poisoning, aspirin poisoning, diabetes, acidic pH in blood, kidney/liver disease, ketoacidosis, ethylene glycol poisoning, lactic acidosis, fever

- FALSE LOW: chlorothiazide diuretics

- Ways to improve your results: CO_2 is increased with alkalinity (e.g., sodium bicarbonate, minerals), decrease with acidity.

- Helpful nutrients: Add a digestive enzyme, lemon water, and super "green" foods.

- See Complete Metabolic Blood Panel in the Appendix.

Carbon Monoxide (CO) (0-15%)

Carbon monoxide is a common gas given off during incomplete combustion (from automobile engines, cigarettes, lawn mowers, household heaters) and is highly toxic because it binds to hemoglobin in the blood. CO is not a normal gas in the human body.

- HIGH: carbon monoxide poisoning can cause an array of toxic effects on the body (e.g., coma can be induced at levels approaching 50%, children and adults with anemia, thyroid dysfunction and angina)

- Ways to improve your results: Excessive CO exposure may be better accomplished by practicing safe measures, including not running the car when inside a garage that is attached to the house, checking the battery of an in-home CO detector, having a qualified technician check your heating system yearly, never heat your home with a gas oven, and do not burn anything in the fireplace or stove that is not properly vented.

Carcinoembryonic Antigen (CEA) (0- 2.5 mcg/ml)

The CEA test measures the level of carcinoembryonic antigen (CEA) in the blood. CEA is a protein normally found in the tissue of a developing baby in the womb. The blood level of this protein disappears or becomes very low after birth. In adults, an abnormal level of CEA may be a sign of cancer.

- HIGH: benign tumors, cancer (of lung), inflammatory disease (colitis, pancreatitis), liver disease, lung infections, ulcers, heavy smokers, gall bladder malfunction

- LOW-NORMAL: expected

- Note: see Cancer Antigen CA-125 and CA-15-3

- See Cancer Serum Tests in the Appendix.

Cardio C-Reactive Protein (CRP) (<1 mg-10.0 mg/L) (for ages over 17 years)

CRP stands for "C-reactive protein" which is made by the liver in response tissue injury, infection and/or inflammation. A desirable cardio CRP is less than 1 mg/L. Increased heart risk is associated with cardio CRP levels exceeding 3 mg/L. When a cardio CRP is above 10 mg/L, risk analysis may be confused by a recent infection or illness. Repeat test in 2 weeks. Frequently other tests are needed to determine the exact site of the inflammatory response.

The inflammatory signaled by CRP is influenced by genetics, a sedentary lifestyle, too much stress, and exposure to environmental toxins such as secondhand tobacco smoke. Diet has a huge impact, particularly one that contains a lot of refined, processed and manufactured foods.

- Low risk: less than 1.0 mg/L
- Average risk: 1.0 to 3.0 mg/L
- High risk: above 3.0 mg/L

- HIGH: infection (viral or bacterial), auto-immune disease (practically all of them), cancer, long-term illness, heart disease, Lyme disease

- LOW: favorable, little concern

- Ways to improve your results (to lower): Eat a non-inflammatory diet (less animal protein, fats, dairy, wheat), exercise, lose weight, increase foods high in antioxidants,

- Helpful nutrients: a potent multi-vitamin-mineral formula, Co-enzyme Q10, L-carnitine, omega-3 fatty acids, vitamin D, vitamins E & C, magnesium, alpha-lipoic acid, omega 7 (palmitoleic acid), L-arginine, selenium, vitamin B-complex, inositol, lecithin, potassium

- Helpful herbs: turmeric (curcumin), grape seed extract, pycnogenol, red yeast rice, garlic, alfalfa, cayenne, green tea, cordyceps, hawthorn, wild oregano, essential oils (e.g., frankincense, melaleuca, lavender, eucalyptus)

- See Cardiac Function Tests in the Appendix.

Catecholamines: Norepinephrine (0-600pg/ml) Epinephrine (0-900)

Catecholamines are biologically active compounds that play key roles in metabolism and cardiovascular function. These simple, structurally similar organic compounds also play vital roles in regulating the function of our nervous systems, both central and peripheral. Without them, our bodies would be like the Internet if all the transmission lines failed—dead. One catecholamine in particular, noradrenaline is involved in mood regulation.

Catecholamines are obtained exclusively by synthesis from nutrient molecules—mainly the amino acids phenylalanine and tyrosine—in our foods. In normal metabolism, phenylalanine converts to tyrosine, which converts via dopa to the catecholamine dopamine; dopamine is the immediate precursor of noradrenaline, which converts to adrenaline. Catecholamines are released into the blood (from the adrenal glands) when a person is under physical or emotional stress.

The main catecholamines are dopamine, adrenalin, epinephrine and norepinephrine. They are metabolized via an oxidizing enzyme in the heart.

- HIGH: acute anxiety, ganglioblastoma (very rare), neuroblastoma (rare), pheochromocytoma (rare), severe stress

- FALSE HIGH: acetaminophen, cocaine, caffeine, amphetamines, albuterol, some anti-depressants

- LOW: depression, age-related mental problems, low mood

- Ways to improve your results (for low levels): Supplement with phenylalanine and other amino acids.

CD-57 Lyme test (60-360)

Drs. Stricker and Winger were involved in the discovery of the CD57 blood test and its relation to Lyme disease. It is often called the "Stricker CD57 panel." CD57+ markers can also be expressed on other kinds of cells, including T-cells and natural-killer (NK) cells.

For a Lyme patient, a normal level of 200 before stopping antibiotics is desired. Lyme disease is a bacterial infection *(Borrelia burgdorferi)* you get from the bite of an infected tick. Lyme is a multi-stage disease caused by a spirochete (another disease-causing germ) transmitted by the tick bite (most commonly a deer tick).

The first symptom is usually a rash, which may look like a bull's eye. As the infection spreads symptoms such as fever, headache, muscle and joint aches, a stiff neck and fatigue can occur over weeks, months and years. Lyme disease can be hard to diagnose because you may not have noticed a tick bite. Blood tests are notoriously inaccurate in giving negative results.

While antibiotics and other prescription meds are certainly helpful in treating the tick-borne infections, experts in natural medicine say there's also a place for holistic remedies in treatment and management.

- HIGH: not significant

- LOW: a test below 60 indicates very active Lyme disease, can be related to all tick-borne diseases

- Ways to improve your results: Homeopathy, consume more "green drinks" to provide chlorophyll for better detoxification.

- Helpful nutrients: Since Lyme may deplete vitamin D, zinc, B-complex, supplement with a multi-vitamin formula, pancreatic enzymes, vitamin C, vitamin A, vitamin E, selenium, omega-3 fatty acids.

- Helpful herbs: wild oregano, wild curcumin, probiotics, chaga mushrooms, garlic, echinacea, goldenseal, alfalfa, dandelion

- Note: See a qualified practitioner before beginning any treatment. See Antibody Serum Tests in the Appendix.

Chloride, Serum (98-110 mEq/L)

Chloride (Cl-) is an electrolyte mineral involved water balance (acid-base) in body fluids. Chloride's main source (sodium chloride) is the diet.

- HIGH (Hyperchloremia): adrenal gland over-activity, aldosterone hormone excess, dehydration, kidney disease, Cushing's disease, metabolic acidosis, multiple myeloma, diabetes, primary hyperparathyroidism, atrial fibrillation, adrenal gland dysfunction

- FALSE HIGH: high altitude, excessive exercise, heavy, rapid breathing, high salt intake, estrogens, androgens, corticosteroids

- LOW (Hypochloremia): may occur in cardiac heart disease, adrenal gland under-activity (Addison's disease), severe vomiting, gastric suction, infections, diabetes, intestinal obstruction, kidney failure, burns, nausea, vomiting

- FALSE LOW: laxative, bicarbonate, diuretics

- Ways to improve your health (if low): Add more tablet salt or sea salt to diet, keep hydrated, avoid alcohol and caffeine (may cause electrolyte disturbances), balance pH level.

- Ways to improve your results (if high): Keep hydrated and avoid alcohol and caffeine (may cause electrolyte disturbances).

- See Adrenal Function Tests, Kidney Renal Function Tests and Pregnancy Serum Tests in the Appendix.

Cholesterol, Total Serum (<200 mg/dL)

Cholesterol is a waxy fat like substance that is important for normal body functioning. Cholesterol is an important lipid that compromises part of the cell membrane and myelin sheath and plays a role in nerves function and the production of hormones.

Your body will produce enough cholesterol to maintain normal body needs. The liver is the major production factory for cholesterol (about 70%).
Levels:
High: >240
Borderline: 200-239
Acceptable: <200 mg/dL

- HIGH: is a strong indicator of the potential for cardiovascular disease, the formation of plaque in the arteries (atherosclerosis)

- LOW: it must be recognized that very low cholesterol levels can be detrimental. Levels under <140 may enhance unnecessary risks (e.g., depression, low libido, muscle weakness, memory loss, dementia, prostate problems in men)

- Ways to improve your results: Consume foods lower in cholesterol (found in the livers of animals), reduce consumption of animal protein, and consume a more plant-based diet.

- Helpful nutrients (to lower): niacin, niacinamide, vitamin E, vitamin C, pantethine, B-complex, alpha-lipoic acid, CoQ10, apple pectin, omega-3 fatty acids, flaxseed, lecithin, buckwheat and pea protein

- Helpful herbs: gugulipids, garlic, hawthorn, red yeast rice, plant sterols, artichoke, curcumin, cinnamon, medical mushrooms, lemongrass essential oil

- See Cardiac Function Tests, Liver/Gall Bladder Individual Function Tests and Pregnancy Serum Tests in the Appendix.

Chlolesterol/HDL Ratio (<4.0)

The total cholesterol to HDL ratio is determined by dividing the total cholesterol number by the HDL number. For most people, the goal is to be below 4.0, with an ideal below 3.4 (men) and 3.3 (women). It should be noted that doctors are divided on the effectiveness of this ratio to predict the chances of developing heart disease.

- HIGH: risk of coronary heart disease, heart attack, stroke, atherosclerosis

- LOW: preferable

- Ways to improve your results: Eat a more plant-based diet.

- Note: See Cholesterol and HDL.

Coagulation Factors

Normal coagulation factor activity usually means normal clotting function. Low activity of one or more coagulation factors usually means impaired clotting ability. Deficiencies in coagulation factors may be acquired (due to other diseases) or inherited, mild or severe, permanent or temporary. Lyme disease may cause an increase in coagulability.

Coagulation Panel (Blood clot retraction)

- Fibrinogen
- PTT
- Platelet count
- Pro time
- Vitamin K
- See Liver/Gall Bladder Individual Function Tests in the Appendix.

Complete Metabolic Panel (CMP)

The CMP is used as a broad screening tool to evaluate organ function and check for conditions such as diabetes, liver and kidney disease. The CMP may also be ordered to monitor known conditions, such as hypertension, and to monitor people taking specific medications for any kidney- or liver-related side effects

- See Complete Metabolic Blood Panel in the Appendix.

Copper, serum (70-155 ng/100ml)

Copper testing is primarily used to help diagnose Wilson disease, a rare inherited disorder that can lead to excess storage of copper in the liver, brain and other organs. Copper is an essential mineral that is stored in muscles and the liver.

In excess, copper can cause toxicity (copperiedus), which refers to the consequences of eating acid foods cooked in uncoated copper cookware, from exposure to copper in drinking water via copper-coated pipes and other environmental sources.

- HIGH: nausea, anemia, heart attack, death, infection, leukemia, jaundice, fatigue, tremors, behavioral changes, dystonia, insomnia, emotionalism, schizophrenia, oligophenia, Tourette's syndrome, bipolar disease, autism

- FALSE HIGH: birth control pills

- LOW: consult physician - may be serious complications: osteoporosis, anemia, neutropenia

- Ways to improve your results (if low): Consume foods that are good sources of copper (e.g., liver, beans, peas, avocado, whole grains, seafood).

- Helpful nutrients (if low): Copper can be supplemented if levels are low (see qualified practitioner), possible depletion of vitamin C, B-complex, manganese and molybdenum.

- Helpful nutrients (if high): It is necessary to supplement with extra zinc to offset copper toxicity and reduce consumption of high copper foods.

- Note: Detoxification methods may be helpful.

Cortisol (Hydrocortisone) (4-19 mcg/dL)

A hormone produced by the adrenals (from cholesterol) and is essential in breaking down fat, sugar and protein. Cortisol also regulates the body's potassium/sodium balance. The adrenals secrete cortisol in response to stress, tension, anxiety, inflammation and infection.

Interleukin IL-6 pays a role in a cortisol-driven response. IL-6 is produced in the immune cells and stimulates the central and sympathetic nervous system, leading to high blood pressure and autonomic imbalance.

- HIGH: Cushing's disease (over secretion of the adrenal gland), TNF-alpha increase which blocks the action of insulin (e.g. metabolic syndrome, liver gluconeogenesis, fatty acid liberation, contributes to weight gain, negatively affects amino acids, and may induce inflammation)

- LOW: Addison's disease, pituitary gland malfunction, adrenal infection or atrophy of adrenal cortex, excess androgen

- FALSE HIGH/LOW: birth control pills, anticonvulsant drugs, estrogen, diuretic, obesity, pregnancy, severe long-term stress

- Ways to improve your results: Adrenal nutrients help balance cortisol levels (high or low), lower IL-6.

- Helpful nutrients (to balance levels): vitamin C, B-complex (B1,B2,B5), folic acid, alpha-lipoic acid, vitamin A, vitamin D, bioflavonoids, magnesium, zinc, vitamin B6, amino acids, chromium, raw adrenal glandular, L-tyrosine

- Helpful herbs (to balance levels): panax ginseng, turmeric, licorice, Mexican yam, astragalus, basil and rosemary essential oils

- See Adrenal Function Tests in the Appendix.

Creatinine (women: 0.5-1.10 mg/dL) (men: 0.6-1.6 mg/dL)

Creatinine is a waste product by the body when creatine, a metabolism substance that helps convert food into energy, breaks down. Usually, your kidneys help filter creatinine out of the blood and the waste product is then passed out of the body via urine. High creatinine indicates a problem with your kidneys and is the most commonly used indicator of kidney function.

- HIGH: muscular dystrophy, decrease in kidney dysfunction (nephritis), long-term diabetes, extensive hypertension, shock

- FALSE HIGH: antibiotic overuse, sedatives, barbiturates, high-dose vitamin C

- LOW: an extremely low protein diet, liver disease, decreased muscle mass (cachexia)

- FALSE LOW: pregnancy, some BP drugs
  Ways to improve your results (to lower): Drink more water to increase creatinine. Eat a vegetarian diet.

- Helpful herbs (to lower): stinging nettles, dandelion, chamomile tea, Siberian ginseng, chitosan, cinnamon, astragalus, ASEA

- Note: Tthe upper reference limit for creatinine in approximately 13% higher for people identified as African-American.

- See Kidney Renal Function Tests and Pregnancy Serum Tests in the Appendix.

Creatinine Phosphokinase (CPK) (10 - 120 mcg/L)

A heart enzyme also found in the liver, brain and skeletal muscle. Since each of these enzymes are slightly different, isolating each CPK "isoenzyme" can help to discover which heart muscle might be damaged. High levels imply that the kidneys are not filtering properly.

- HIGH: When the total CPK level is very high, it usually means there has been injury or stress to muscle tissue, heart or brain. This can include a heart attack, heart muscle inflammation, heart injury, muscular dystrophy, brain injury, stroke, convulsions, electrical shock

- FALSE HIGH: excessive alcohol intake, high protein diet, strenuous exercise

- LOW: of no importance

- Ways to improve your results: Eat foods that lower blood pressure and cholesterol, including artichoke, legumes, almonds and walnuts (Mediterranean diet).

- Helpful nutrients: omega-3-fatt acids, magnesium, vitamins A and C
- Helpful herbs: ashwagandha, ginkgo biloba, garlic, red yeast rice
- See Cardiac Function Tests and Kidney Renal Function Tests in the Appendix.

Cyclic Citrulline PEP IgG (CCP) (<20 Units)

The CCP test is used to evaluate patients suspected of having rheumatoid arthritis (RA). Cyclic Citrulline PEP may differentiate rheumatoid arthritis from other connective tissue diseases that may present with arthritis. Rheumatoid arthritis (RA) is a systemic autoimmune disease characterized by chronic joint inflammation that ultimately leads to joint destruction. RA affects approximately 1% of the world's population. Underlying causes of RA could include glute intolerance, mercury or heavy metals poisoning, mycotoxins, leaky-gut syndrome and infection.

- Low (negative): <20 units indicates no CCP IgG antibodies present, little concern
- Weak (positive): 20-39 units, semi-quantitative
- Moderate (positive): 40-59 units indicates the presence of CCP IgG antibodies
- High (strong positive): > 59 levels
- Ways to improve your results: Remove gluten from your diet, treat infections if present, test for heavy metals, heal the gut, support the immune system.
- Helpful nutrients: borage oil, fish oil, probiotics
- Helpful herbs: turmeric, boswellia, ginger, essential oils (e.g., marjoram, lavender, cypress, geranium)
- Note: See ANA test, Sed rate, ESR, RF and Cardio CRP.

Dehydroepiandrosterone (DHEA) (19-321 mcg/dL)

DHEA sulfate is the most abundant hormone found in the bloodstream produced by the adrenal gland in both men and women. The DHEA sulfate test is often done in women who have male body characteristics (e.g., virilism, excessive hair growth, irregular periods or infertility). It may also be done in women with pituitary disease or adrenal disease who are concerned about low libido or decreased sexual satisfaction.

If you live to be 80, your body will probably have only 10-20% of the DHEA you had when you were 20 years old. The healthiest older humans usually have higher levels of DHEA levels, while the sickest individuals have the lowest levels. High and low levels are not generally recognized as a medical condition; it usually indicates the need for further testing.

- HIGH: associated with Cushing disease, adrenal cancer, andrenocortical tumor, adrenal hyperplasia

- LOW: adrenal insufficiency, adrenal dysfunction, atherosclerotic plaque, nerve degeneration, Addison's disease, hypopituitarism, vulnerability to breast, prostate and bladder cancer

- Ways to improve your results (to increase): Research suggests that DHEA replacement therapy can have a number of highly beneficial effects (e.g., increased lifespan, inhibit the proliferation of cancer cells, enhanced immune system and preventing osteoporosis in women).

- Ways to improve your results (to lower): It is more difficult to do but try taking birth control pills, lose weight if obese, and/or take extra vitamin E.

- Note: DHEA therapy should be undertaken with caution; see a qualified practitioner before beginning replacement therapy.

- Helpful nutrients: DHEA along with vitamin C, vitamin E, selenium

- See Adrenal Function Tests, DHEA Normal Serum Levels and Estrogen Dominance in the Appendix.

Estimated Glomerular Follicle Rate (eGFR) (90-120 ml/min)

eGFR is an estimated rate, usually based on serum creatinine level, age, sex, and race. eGFR is used to screen for and detect early kidney damage and to monitor kidney status. It is performed by ordering a creatinine test and calculating the estimated glomerular filtration rate. eGFR has a significant meaning for people with kidney disease, especially advanced kidney disease. It also has been used to estimate how much blood passes through the tiny filters of the kidney (called glomeruli) each minute. If your eGFR value is lower than the normal (100 ml/min-140 ml/min), it indicates that your kidney isn't functioning optimally. If the eGFR continues to fall, kidney dialysis may be evident.

eGFR is only an estimate so significant error is possible. eGFR is most likely to be inaccurate in people at extremes of body type; for example, malnourished, amputees, certain races, pregnant women, children, etc. See Glomerular Filtration Rate (GFR).

- eGFR Caucasian/other American: (> or = to 60 ml/min/1.73m2)
- eGFR African American: (> or = to 60 ml/min/1.73m2. African American age 60-69 (85 ml/min/1.73m2)
- eGFR<100 ml/min may indicate moderate kidney dysfunction
- eGFR<60 ml/min indicates kidney disease
- eGFR<15 ml/min indicates kidney failure
- LOW: factors likely to damage kidney function (e.g., heart disease, hypertension, diabetes, family history, excessive bleeding, frequent urinary infections) can cause low eGFR levels
- Ways to improve things naturally (to raise): Eat a more vegetarian diet, consult a nutritionist regarding a high- versus low-protein diet, water hydration, juicing, traditional Chinese medicine, exercise.

THE BLOOD TESTS

- See Kidney Renal Function Tests in the Appendix.

Electrolytes, serum

Electrolytes are the charged particles in the body fluid that hold and conduct electricity. When these particles are properly combined (positive and negative particles), the fluid will be "electrically neutral", thereby accounting for better pH balance.

- HIGH/LOW: Depending on which electrolyte is out of balance and the extent of that change, treatment may involve a change in diet (e.g., lower salt intake, decrease fluid intake, balance acid-alkaline level, take medications for balance).

- FALSE HIGH: drugs such as anabolic steroids, laxatives, oral contraceptives, cortisone

- FALSE LOW: diuretics, carbamazepine, tricyclic antidepressants.

- Note: See individual serum electrolytes: calcium, chloride, magnesium, potassium, sodium, and sodium bicarbonate.

Eosinophils, Absolute (0.0-0.4 109 cells/L) (0-400 cells/mcL) (1-4%)

An absolute eosinophil count is a blood test that measures the number of a type of white blood cell (WBC) called eosinophils. Eosinophils become active when you have certain allergic diseases, mold, and especially parasites. One third of body's histamine is found here.

These eosinophils, also known as granulocytes, are developed during the formation of blood cellular components in the bone marrow, whereupon they migrate into the blood. On average, 5-7% of the white blood cells are constituents of eosinophils. High counts are considered and eosinophilia disease. Eosinophils are a kind of bronchitis, which causes inflammation of the airways and can result in coughing and difficult breathing and a need for further testing.

- HIGH: asthma, allergies such as hay fever, food allergies, parasitic infections, inflammatory disorders (e.g., IBS, celiac, disease), leukemia or Hodgkin's lymphomas, hay fever, eczema, skin disorders, immunodeficiency

- FALSE HIGH: interferon, tranquilizers, certain antibiotics, some laxatives (psyllium), amphetamines

- Note: High levels usually indicate a need for further testing.

- LOW: alcohol intoxication, steroids long-term use, Cushing's disease (acute renal failure), acute bacterial infections

- Ways to improve your results (to stabilize levels): Yoga, vegetarian diet, alkaline pH, exercise, relaxation and anything that enhances immune function.

- Helpful nutrients (to lower allergic reaction): omega-3-fatty acids, quercetin, vitamin C, acidophilus, beta-1,3 glucan, Coenzyme Q10, acetyl-L-carnitine

- Helpful herbs: stinging nettles, turmeric (curcumin), neem, licorice, ashwagandha, wild oregano, holy basil, ginger, fenugreek seeds, eucalyptus oil

- Note: If parasites are determined, consider supplementing with homeopathy, garlic, colloidal silver, anti-parasitic formulas and essential oils (e.g., oregano, thyme, fennel, chamomile, melaleuca)

- Note: See a qualified practitioner before treating parasitic infections.

- See Antibody Serum Tests in the Appendix.

Estradiol, serum (E2) (premenopausal women 15-350 pg/ml) (post-menopausal women <10 pg/ml) (men 10-40 pg/ml)

Estradiol (E2) is produced primarily in the ovaries and testes by the aromatization of testosterone. Small amounts are produced in the adrenal glands and some peripheral tissue, mostly fat.

Measurement of serum E2 forms an integral part of the assessment of function of the female reproductive organs, including assessment of fertility, amenorrhea and menopausal status. It is widely used for monitoring ovulation induction, as well as during preparation for in-vitro fertilization. After menopause, estradiol production drops to a very low but constant level.

- HIGH: hypogonadism (check LH and FSH levels), polycystic ovarian syndrome (PCOS), androgen producing tumors, ovarian producing tumors, cancer, early puberty, cirrhosis, hyperthyroidism, estrogen dominance, diseases of the hypothalamus or pituitary glands

- FALSE HIGH: could be functional causes such as starvation, over exercise, severe emotional and/or physical stress, excess drug and/or alcohol use

- LOW: anti-estrogen therapy, low bone density, delayed puberty, low pituitary function, anti-androgen therapy in men

- Ways to improve your results: See a qualified health practitioner and investigate in bioidentical hormone replacement.

- Helpful nutrients (if low): flaxseed, chasteberry, foods high in phytoestrogens

- Note: Estradiol is the most potent and most carcinogenic.

- See Adrenal Function Tests and Estrogen Dominance in the Appendix.

Estriol, serum (E3) (adult female <.21 ng/ml)
(adult male <.18 ng/ml)(pregnancy varies from 2.50-14.60 mg/ml)

A female hormone produced in large amounts by the placenta (the tissue that links the fetus to the mother) during pregnancy. It can be detected as early as the 9th week of pregnancy and its levels increase until delivery.

Estriol is a safer form of estrogen because it isn't metabolized into other hormones; it's a one-way street. It never loses its unique identity. Estriol does not have the potential to damage DNA and initiate cancer like its sister estrogens, estradiol and estrone. While estriol is not capable of initiating cancer, it can stimulate the growth of a preexisting cancer if the estriol concentration is high enough. Whether or not estriol stimulates breast cancer cell growth depends on the dose, timing and delivery system.

- HIGH: multiple fetuses

- NORMAL: steadily rises throughout pregnancy

- LOW: adrenal problems, anemia, diabetes, hypertension, kidney and/or liver disease, malnutrition

- Ways to improve your results: Check for possible low levels of vitamins B6 and B12.

- Helpful nutrients (if low): flaxseed, chasteberry, foods high in phytoestrogens

- Note: Estriol comprises nearly 80% of the total free estrogen in the female body.

- See Adrenal Function Tests and Estrogen Dominance in the Appendix.

Estrone, serum (E1) (pre-menopausal women 17-200 pg/ml) (post-menopausal women 7-40 pg/ml) (men 10-60 pg/ml)

Estrogen tests are used to detect a deficiency or excess in a woman and to help diagnose a variety of conditions associated with this imbalance. They may also be used to help determine the timing of a woman's ovulation and may be ordered to monitor the health status of the developing baby and placenta during pregnancy.

Estrone is produced and more predominant during menopause and may be measured in women who have gone through menopause to determine their estrogen levels. Estrone is 70% less biologically active than estradiol (E2). Estrone is a significant estrogenic hormone in both reproductive and post-menopausal women and in men. It may be tested in women who might have cancer of the ovaries, testicles or adrenal glands. In a man, estrogen testing may be performed to detect a hormone excess and its cause (e.g., testicle cancer).

- HIGH: polycystic ovarian syndrome (PCOS), androgen producing tumors, ovarian producing tumors, may cause damage fertility or the unborn child. In men, cancer and heart disease.

- LOW: anti-estrogen therapy, low bone density, delayed puberty

- Ways to improve your results (to lower): Eat organic foods, exercise more, limit dairy products, decrease alcohol intake and eat more fiber.

- Helpful nutrients (to raise): flaxseed, chasteberry, foods high in phytoestrogens

- See Adrenal Function Tests and Estrogen Dominance in the Appendix.

Ferritin (33-232 ng/ml)

Ferritin is a cellular and intracellular protein that binds, stores and releases iron in a safe form. Ferritin is the best indicator of the amount of uncommitted iron reserves and identifies the amount of iron in the blood. A series of falling dominos occurs with lower ferritin levels. There is a hidden connection between ferritin levels and liver function that needs to be more investigated.

- HIGH: possible infection, iron overload, leukemia, liver disease, autoimmunity, Lyme disease

- LOW: anemia from iron deficiency, digestive tract bleeding, heavy menstruation, unexplained rash on the body, intestinal and/or liver imbalance, overgrowth of Candida albicans, overuse of antibiotics, synthetic chemical toxicity, hypothyroidism, excessive exercise (e.g., long-distance runners)

- FALSE LOW: excessive alcohol consumption

- Ways to improve your results (to increase): Consume more iron-rich foods to raise the level, avoid extensive use of antibiotics and be careful of foods that contain higher levels of antibiotics (i.e. poultry, ground meats, sausage, and hamburgers). Begin consuming fermented foods like miso, kombucha and plain goat's milk yogurt.

- Note: Taking too many iron pills can be counter-productive (when ferritin is low).

- Helpful Nutrients: probiotics (Lactobacillus acidophilus), prebiotics, essential fatty acids

Fibrinogen (150-350 mg/dL)

Fibrinogen is a protein (along with thrombin) produced by the liver that helps to stop bleeding by helping in the formation of blood clots. This test is performed on patients with bleeding disorders

- HIGH: acute infections, cancer, heart disease, MI, vitamin K deficiency, trauma. Higher levels may also increase the risk of blood clots leading to cardiovascular disease.

- LOW: end-stage liver disease, bone cancer, vitamin B deficiency, malnutrition, blood transfusion

- Ways to improve your results: Improving levels are akin to decreasing the risk of stroke and hardening of the arteries (e.g., eat healthy, minimize calcium intake, maximize magnesium intake).

- Helpful nutrients (to lower): vitamin K2, vitamin D3, amino acids, nattokinase, resveratrol, barley grass

Folic Acid (Folate) (Vitamin B4) (5-25 ng/ml)

Folic acid (folates are related compounds) is a water-soluble vitamin not produced by the body, but is essential for the body's health. Folic acid is vital for the production of new cells (the building blocks of life) and works with vitamin B12 to abate pernicious anemia. Some scientists also speculate that folic acid plays a role in maintaining heart health and preventing cell mutations that may lead to cancer.

- HIGH: non-toxic but can mask vitamin B12 deficiency

- LOW: blood disease, alcoholism, poor diet, mal-absorption in gut, overactive thyroid

- FALSE LOW: cancer drugs, birth control pills, low vitamin C, diet low in greens and fruits

- Ways to improve your results: For general deficiency, it is best to supplement; see a qualified practitioner for dosage.

- Helpful nutrients: foods high in folate include (e.g., sprouted wheat, bulgur, wheat germ, soybean flour, sun flowers, black-eyed peas, raw potatoes)

- Helpful herbs: kelp, ginseng, feverfew, hops, slippery elm, spirulina (blue-green algae)

Follicle Stimulating Hormone (FSH) (women: before puberty 0-5.0 mIU/ml) (during puberty 0.3-10.0 mIU/ml) (menstruating 4.7-21.5 IU/ml) (after menopause 25.8-134.8 mIU/ml) (men: before or during puberty (0-10.0 mIU/ml) (adult male: 1.5-12.4 mIU/ml)

The FSH blood test measures the level of FSH in blood. FSH is a hormone released by the pituitary gland, located on the underside of the brain. In women, FSH helps control the menstrual cycle and the production of eggs by the ovaries. The amount of FSH varies throughout a woman's menstrual cycle and is highest just before she releases an egg (ovulates). In men, FSH helps control the production of sperm. The amount of FSH in men normally remains constant.

- HIGH (women): during or after menopause, including premature menopause, when receiving hormone therapy, tumor in the pituitary gland, Turner's syndrome

- HIGH (men): advancing age (male menopause), damage to testicles (from chemotherapy or radiation), treatment with hormones, tumors in the pituitary gland

- LOW (women): pregnancy, being very underweight, not ovulating, the pituitary gland or hypothalamus not producing normal amounts of some or all of its hormones; (men) low sperm count

- Ways to improve your results (to raise FSH): Consume more omega-3 fatty acids, eat alkalizing foods and reduce stress (yoga).

- Ways to improve results (to lower FSH): Consult with a specialist about trying certain Chinese herbs.

- Helpful nutrients (to balance): B-complex, CoenzymeQ-10

- Helpful herbs (to raise): ginseng, vitex, maca, saw palmetto, tribulus

- See Estrogen Dominance in the Appendix.

Free Thyroxine Index (FTI) (4.6-10.9 mg/dL)

FTI measures the amount of T4 (thyroxine) circulating in the blood (not stored) and hence available for metabolic activity. This is a test of thyroid metabolism calculated by multiplying the level of T4 times the level of T3 uptake = FTI.

- HIGH: thyroid hyper-function

- LOW: obesity, possible diabetes

- Ways to improve your results: The way we eat can actually help or hurt our thyroid gland. The nutrients our thyroid needs are easily accessible in many foods and dietary supplements.

- Helpful nutrients: selenium, vitamin D3, probiotics, iodine (under supervision)
- Note: See TSH, T3, T4.
- See Thyroid Function Tests in the Appendix.

Galactose Transferase (GALT) (> or = 24.5 nmol/mg of homeglobin)

Galactose is a simple monosaccharide that serves as an energy source and as an essential component of glycolipids and glycoproteins. Galactose transferase is an enzyme that breaks down sugar galactose (in milk, sugar beets, seaweed). Without the enzyme, damage can result to the eyes, liver, kidneys and tissues—a disorder called galactosemia. Low levels may risk learning and speech disabilities, ovarian failure, tremors.

- HIGH: patients with higher levels of residual enzyme activity can typically tolerate higher levels of galactose in their diets
- LOW: there is no cure for galactose deficiency, in the most severely affected patients; treatment involves a galactose free diet for life
- Ways to improve your results: Eliminate all lactose (milk sugar) and galactose from the diet.
- Note: Early identification and implementation of a modified diet improves patient outcomes.
- Helpful nutrients: after diagnosis, patients who are deficient are often supplemented with calcium, magnesium and extra vitamin D

Gamma Globulins (2-3 gm/dL)

A gamma globulin test is used to test the amount of immunoglobins in the blood. Immunoglobins are also called immune gamma globulins. Immunoglobins are antibodies that are produced by the body in response to foreign substances, such as bacteria, viruses and cancerous cells. Gamma globulin is a protein in the blood plasma that keeps infections and disease at bay, acting in tandem with our antibodies to keep us healthy. Thus maintaining the right level of gamma globulin levels is necessary for healthy living. (See Immunoglobulins.)

Gamma Glutamyl Transferase (GGT) (2-65 U/L)

GGT is an enzyme produced by the bile ducts in the liver and muscles. It contributes to the breakdown of fat. The (GGT) test may be used to determine the cause of elevated alkaline phosphatase (ALP). This usually occurs when liver damage or disease is suspected.

- HIGH: liver disease (hepatitis, cirrhosis) and chronic alcoholism
- HIGH (Moderate): diabetes, chronic heart disease, gall bladder, and pancreatitis.
- LOW or NORMAL: little indication of any liver disease, hypothyroidism
- Ways to improve your results: Eating more fruits and vegetables can lower GGT, as can consumption of quality protein (e.g., whey, eggs, poultry). These foods contain the amino acid cysteine.
- Helpful nutrients: the nutrient glutathione and extra antioxidants can reduce oxidative stress (e.g., environmental toxins, radiation, pesticides, heavy metals, e-smog)
- See Cardiac Function Tests and Liver/Gall Bladder Individual Function Tests in the Appendix.

Gastrin (0-700 pg/ml)

Gastrin is a peptide hormone that stimulates secretion of gastric acid (HCl) by the parietal cells of the stomach and aids in gastric motility, gall bladder function and maturation of food. It is released by G cells in the pyloric antrum of the stomach, duodenum and pancreas.

- HIGH: anemia, gastric problems, ulcers, cancer, kidney disease, hypoglycemia

- FALSE LOW: alcohol, high amino acid intake, H-2 drugs (Zantac, Pepcid), protein pump inhibitor drugs (Prilosec, Prevacid), eating before the exam

- Ways to improve your results: Take a multi-digestive enzyme (containing gastrin) 5 to 15 minutes before larger meals for improved digestion and gastric emptying.

Glomerular Filtration Rate (GFR) (90-120 ml/min)

GFR is used to check how well the kidneys are working. Creatinine is not sensitive to early renal (kidney) damage since it varies with age, gender and/or ethnicity. The impact of these variables can be reduced by estimating GFR. GFR estimates how much blood passes through the tiny filters of the kidneys each minute.

- HIGH: increased during pregnancy

- LOW: levels below 60 ml/min for 3 months is a sign of chronic kidney disease, below 15 ml/min indicates kidney failure

- Ways to improve your results: Difficult to do, but GFR may be slightly raised with exercise, juicing (organic vegetables), limiting animal protein and salt intake, sunshine, relaxation, asparagus.

- Helpful nutrients: vitamin D, alkaline powder

- Helpful herbs (to raise): milk thistle, goldenrod, dandelion root, horsetail, celery root, uva-ursi, essential oils (e.g., lemongrass, thyme, juniper berry, grapefruit)

- See Kidney Renal Function Tests in the Appendix.

Glucocorticoids

Glucocorticoids are adrenal gland steroid hormones that influence protein and carbohydrate metabolism. These are necessary in stress conditions, such as pregnancy. They regulate the production of sugar from protein when blood sugar drops (hypoglycemia), and control the loss of potassium from tissues that creates insulin resistance to enhance white blood cell effort. Cortisol (or hydrocortisone) is the most important human glucocorticoid.

- HIGH: Cushing's syndrome, chronic disease
- LOW: severe hypertension, infectious disease, surgery, burns, pancreatitis, rheumatoid arthritis
- Ways to improve your results: Supplementing with amino acids may help the transport of glucocorticoids.
- Note: Levels can be affected by heavy metal toxins. See Cortisol.

Glucose (65-99 mg/dL)

The blood glucose level is the amount of glucose (sugar) present in the blood of a human or animal. Glucose is a by-product of carbohydrate digestion (processed via the pancreas) and is used as an immediate source of energy or stored as fat for later use (glycogen). The human body naturally tightly regulates blood glucose levels as a part of metabolic homeostasis.

- HIGH: diabetes, pre-diabetes, hypertension, liver disease, infectious disease, over-activity of endocrine system, carbon monoxide poisoning, central nervous system disease
- LOW: inability to store glucose, liver disease, pancreatic disease, under-activity of endocrine system, starvation, poor diet
- Ways to improve your levels (to lower blood glucose): Increase exercise, improve sleep, drink unsweetened green tea, avoid

consumption of refined carbohydrates and excess animal protein.

- Helpful nutrients: GTF chromium, zinc, magnesium, vanadium, vitamin C, niacin, L-carnitine, omega-3 fatty acids

- Helpful herbs: cinnamon, stevia, gymnema sylvestre, bilberry, bitter melon, aloe vera

- See Cardiac Function Tests, Complete Metabolic Blood Panel, Liver/Gall Bladder Individual Function Tests and Pregnancy Serum Tests in the Appendix.

Glucose Fasting (FBS) (65-99 mg/dL)

Fasting blood sugar (FBS) measures blood glucose for at least 8 hours after you have not eaten. It is often the first test done to check for pre-diabetes and diabetes. Two-hour postprandial blood sugar measures blood glucose exactly 2 hours after you start eating a meal.

- Note: Blood sugar levels can be affected by food or beverages you have ingested recently, your current stress level and medications you may be taking at certain time of the day. This is not a test to measure diabetes.

Glutathione (GSH) (544-1,228 mmol/L)

Glutathione is a powerful endogenous antioxidant (more than 20-30 times the antioxidant effect on vitamins C and E). Glutathione has been the subject of increased scientific interest. Glutathione protects against oxidative stress (the aging process) and ridding the body of free radicals. It is also important in the metabolism and excretion of heavy metals and xenobiotic compounds. Glutathione is a "tripeptide", which means it is composed of three amino acids: glycine, cysteine and glutamic acid. The blood test is not considered highly accurate at this time.

- HIGH: not common

- LOW: coronary artery disease, various types of cancer, asthma, neurodegenerative disorders, cognitive-behavioral problems, autoimmune disorders, normal aging process, liver disease, asthma, cystic fibrosis, stroke, seizures, Alzheimer's disease

- FALSE LOW: alcohol intake, cigarette smoke
  Ways to improve your results: Take oral glutathione in a capsule or liquid (liposomal) form.

- Note: A more absorbable intravenous form is available by licensed practitioners.

- Helpful nutrients: lipoic acid regenerates glutathione, N-acetyl cysteine (NAC) is a glutathione booster

Glycohemoglobin (GHb) (4.5-7.0%)

Glycohemoglobin (also known as glycosylated hemoglobin) is hemoglobin to which glucose is bound, a measure of the long-term control of diabetes mellitus. GHb is increased in the red blood cells of persons with poorly controlled diabetes mellitus. Since the glucose stays attached to hemoglobin for the life of the red blood cell (normally about 120 days), the level of GHb reflects the average blood glucose level.

- HIGH: uncontrolled diabetes mellitus, inadequate diabetes treatment

- FALSE HIGH: laboratory mistakes, high lipid levels, hemoglobin variants

- Note: See Hemoglobin and Cardio HbA1c.

Granulocytes Percentage (0.0-0.1 109 cells/L) (42.2-75.2%)

Granulocytes are a type of white blood cell that is made of small granules, which contain proteins. The types of these cells are neutrophils (mainly), eosinophils and basophils. Granulocytes are immune cells that are filled with toxic granules that are released in the body to target and kill bacteria and viral particles.

- HIGH %: serious infections, bone marrow disorders, autoimmune diseases, neutrophilia

- LOW %: people with lower numbers of granulocytes are more likely to get viral, bacterial infections, chemotherapy, certain cancers, radiation and autoimmune diseases (lower immunity)

- Note: See Neutrophils.

Haptoglobin (41-165 mg/dL)

Haptoglobin is a protein produced by the liver. It attaches to a type of hemoglobin in the blood. Haptoglobin testing is used primarily to help detect and evaluate hemolytic anemia and to distinguish it from anemia due to other causes; however, it cannot be used to diagnose the cause of the hemolysis.

If a haptoglobin level is low or unexpectedly high, then testing may be repeated at a later time to evaluate changes in concentration.

- HIGH: blockage of the bile, joint or muscle inflammation, swelling and pain that comes on suddenly, peptic ulcer, ulcerative colitis, acute myocardial infarction

- FALSE HIGH: corticosteroids, androgens

- LOW: chronic liver disease, collection of blood (hematoma), drug-induced immune hemolytic anemia, blood disorder in a fetus or newborn, anemia, both idiopathic autoimmune and immune hemolytic anemia, liver disease

- FALSE LOW: isoniazid, birth control pills, indomethacin, diphenhydramine

- Ways to improve your results: Consider consuming foods or supplements that will lower the inflammatory response.

- Note: See Globulin.

HDL Cholesterol (>45 mg/dL)

HDL cholesterol is the "good" cholesterol. It is believed that the higher the number, the lower the risk. This is because HDL cholesterol protects against heart disease by taking the "bad" cholesterol (LDL) out of the blood and keeping it away from building up in the arteries. An HDL above 60 md/dL is associated with lower risk of heart disease.

- HIGH: decrease the risk of heart disease

- LOW: lower levels, the greater risk of heart attack, diabetes, bile obstruction, kidney and pancreas disease, underactive thyroid

- Ways to improve your results: Exercise, quit smoking, maintain a stable weight, minimize alcohol, and eliminate consuming trans-fats and saturated fats.

- Helpful nutrients: niacin (niacinamide), inositol, vitamin E

- Helpful herbs: Indian gooseberry, red yeast rice

- Note: See Cholesterol, total serum.

- See Cardiac Function Tests in the Appendix.

Hematocrit (HCT) (women: 37-48%) (men: 45-52%)

This screening measures how much of your blood is made of red blood cells (RBCs). A hematocrit measurement is useful in identifying anemia, bleeding disorders, liver disease, and red cell production within the circulatory system. Hematocrit also shows the oxygen carrying capacity of blood.

- HIGH: bone marrow disorder, blood disease, dengue fever, dehydration, lung disease (COPD), anabolic steroids, shock

- FALSE HIGH: smoking, high altitude

- LOW: low blood oxygen, anemia, hemorrhage, heavy bleeding

with menstruation, Hodgkin's lymphoma, heart failure, chronic kidney disease, leukemia, toxins

- FALSE LOW: vitamin B2, iron folate deficiency

- Ways to improve your results (to raise low hematocrit): Supplement with iron (eat foods high in iron), blood transfusions, IV fluids, folate, vitamin B12, vitamin B6, vitamin A, vitamin C and a potent multi-vitamin-mineral formula.

- Ways to improve your results (to lower high hematocrit): Donate blood, avoid eating meat and drink more water. Check for hyperthyroidism and low testosterone levels.

- See Pregnancy Serum Tests in the Appendix.

Hemoglobin (HgB) (men: 13.5-18 g/dL) (women: 11.7-15.5 g/dL)

HgB is an iron-containing protein that enables RBCs to carry oxygen from the lungs to the rest of the body and excretes carbon dioxide as a waste product. It is composed of heme, which affects the color of RBCs. The amount of HgB determines how much oxygen the RBCs are capable of carrying to other cells.

- HIGH: blood is too thick, over-production of red blood cells, COPD, congestive heart failure (CHF)

- LOW: anemia (various types), bleeding, lead poisoning, malnutrition, over hydration

- Ways to improve your results (to raise): Eat foods high in iron; (to lower) donate blood, vitamin K.

- Helpful nutrients (to raise): vitamins B6, B12, folate, iron and vitamin C

- Helpful herbs (to raise): ashwagandha, dong quai, nettle leaf, chitosan

- Note: The drug Epigen stimulates RBC production.

- See Pregnancy Serum Tests in the Appendix.

Hemoglobin A1C (<5.7%)

The hemoglobin A1c test, also called the HbA1c glycated hemoglobin test, is an important blood test that shows how well your diabetes is being controlled. It develops when hemoglobin, a protein within red blood cells that carries oxygen throughout your body, joins with glucose in the blood, thereby becoming "glycated." Hemoglobin A1c provides an average of your blood sugar control over the past 2 to 3 months. The HbA1c test should be used along with home blood sugar monitoring to make adjustments in your diabetes medications.

- HIGH: diabetes mellitus and the complicated diseases, diabetic retinopathy

- LOW: hypoglycemia (e.g., weakness, cold sweats, hunger in between meals, blurred vision, shakiness, headache)

- Ways to improve your results (to lower): Minimize intake of refined carbohydrates. Get exercise, manage stress and lose weight, if necessary.

- Helpful nutrients (to lower): L-arginine, vanadium, alpha-lipoic acid, chromium, vitamin E, zinc, magnesium, inositol, niacin, biotin, conjugated linoleic acid, digestive enzymes, omega-3 fatty acids

- Helpful herbs (to lower): gymnema sylvestre, maitake mushrooms, bitter melon, pectin, essential oils (e.g., cinnamon, rosemary, geranium, eucalyptus)

- Note: See Glucose.

- See Complete Metabolic Blood Panel in the Appendix.

HLA B-27 Antigen (positive/negative)

Human leukocyte antigen B27 (HLA-B27) is a blood test that identifies a specific protein located on the surface of your white blood cells called human leukocyte antigen B27. Human leukocyte antigens (HLAs) are proteins commonly found on white blood cells. These antigens help your immune system identify differences between healthy body tissue and foreign substances that may cause infection.

Although most HLAs protect the body from harm, HLA-B27 is a specific type of protein that contributes to immune system dysfunction. The presence of HLA-B27 on your white blood cells can cause your immune system to attack the healthy cells that contain it. When this occurs, it can result in an autoimmune disease, such as juvenile rheumatoid disease.

- HIGH (POSITIVE): is associated with a host of autoimmune diseases, including: ankylosing spondylitis (causes inflammation of the bones in the spine), reactive arthritis (causes inflammation of the joints, urethra, and eyes and sometimes lesions on the skin) juvenile rheumatoid arthritis, anterior uveitis

Homocysteine, serum (5.0-20.0 mcmol/L)

Homocysteine is an amino acid used to assess methylation function that is associated with a risk of vascular disease (atherosclerosis, hypertension, cardiovascular disease), cancer and neurological diseases. Homocysteine is a toxic by-product of methionine protein metabolism.

- HIGH: Although uncommon, hereditary could be a factor. Homocysteine levels increase in the body when the metabolism to cysteine of methionine to cysteine is impaired. This may be due to dietary deficiencies in vitamin B6, vitamin B12 and folic acid.

- FALSE HIGH: alcoholism

- LOW: heart attack, stroke, coronary artery disease, hypertension, higher cholesterol, accelerates to the aging process

- FALSE LOW: birth control pills, high fat diets, smoking

- Ways to improve your results (to lower): Methylation is dependent on vitamin B12, niacin, folic acid, vitamin B6, glycine, taurine, betaine and SAMe.

- Note: See a qualified practitioner for dosage.
- See Cardiac Function Tests in the Appendix.

Human Chorionic Gonatropin (HCG) (> 5.0 mlU/ml negative for pregnancy) (>25 mlU/ml positive for pregnancy)

A quantitative human chorionic gonadotropin (HCG) test measures the specific level of HCG in the blood. HCG is a hormone produced in the body during pregnancy (placenta) but also stimulates the testes to produce androgens. In 85% of normal pregnancies, the HCG will double every 48 to 72 hours. As you get further along in the pregnancy the HCL level gets higher. Caution must be used in making too much of the numbers. A normal pregnancy may be low in HCG and have a perfectly normal baby.

- HIGH: multiple pregnancies, ovarian cancer, chloriocarcinoma in the uterus, testicle cancer in men
- LOW: if pregnancy is confirmed and the HCG levels do not rise, there may be a problem with the pregnancy (miscarriage more likely)
- Ways to improve your results: Take a prenatal vitamin formula, omega-3 fatty acids and extra folic acid, iodine (only if levels are low), minerals (magnesium, calcium, potassium and sodium), which may balance all sex hormones involved.
- Note: See a qualified practitioner before proceeding.

Human Growth Hormone (HGH)

Human growth hormone (HGH) testing is primarily used to identify growth hormone deficiency and to help evaluate pituitary gland function, usually as a follow-up to other abnormal pituitary hormone test results. GH testing is also used to detect excess GH and to help diagnose and monitor the treatment of acromegaly and gigantism (abnormal long bone growth). Growth hormone is essential for normal growth and development and helps regulate metabolism in both children and adults. Generally, the pituitary gland makes enough HGH for life. The GH test is also known as the somatotropic hormones test. It requires a 10-12 hour fast.

- GH stimulation testing is ordered for a child when there are signs and symptoms of growth hormone deficiency (GHD), such as a growth rate that slows down in early childhood, shorter stature than other children of the same chronological age, delayed puberty and delayed bone development.

- Note: Use caution as this test has limited value in assessing growth hormone secretion in normal children.

- Helpful nutrients: HGH is activated by amino acids (glycine, tyrosine, glutamine), zinc, niacin, vitamin B6, choline and vitamin C. The homeopathic, herbal and drug forms of HGH are controversial.

Human Papillomavirus (HPV) (Positive/Negative)

More than 70 types of human papillomavirus (HPV) have been identified. They are generally classified as high-risk or low-risk depending on their relationship (or lack of relationship) with cancer and high-grade cervical intraepithelial neoplasia (CIN 2-3). HPV viruses are predominantly sexually transmitted and high-risk HPV types are a major risk factor for the development of cervical cancer. Low-risk HPV types 6 and 11 have been associated with the presence of genital warts or cervical cancer. The HPV virus can be symptoms free.

- Ways to improve your results: Natural treatments include homeopathy and biological medicines, or use other therapies to strengthen the immune system.

- Helpful herbs: shiitake mushrooms, oregano oil, echinacea, goldenseal, turmeric (curcumin), garlic, tea tree oil, pau d'arco, cat's claw, wild oregano

- Note: See a qualified practitioner before taking any supplements that may interfere with accepted drug therapy.

Immunoglobulins Antibodies, serum (mg/ml)

Immunoglobulin antibodies are types of white blood cells made from B-lymphocytes that circulate in the blood and create antibodies that destroy organisms.

There are 5 kinds of antibodies produced by the body: (IgA, IgG, IgM, IgE, and IgD). Each of them helps to protect the body against specific infections and diseases. Low levels can make you more susceptible to diseases.

- IgA (85-385 mg/dL): Antibodies help to protect parts of the body that are exposed to the environment. They are found in the nose, ears, eyes, digestive tract and vagina.

- IgD (<1%): antibodies are found in tissues that line the chest and belly. IgA is found in a very small percentage, and its exact function is yet to be understood completely.

- IgE (<115 Ku/L): These antibodies help in fighting off foreign substances such as pollen, spores, parasites and other antigens. They are found in the lungs, skin and mucous membranes.

- IgG (694-1618 mg/dL): These antibodies help in fighting bacterial and viral infections. They are found in body fluids and may be useful in food allergy testing.

- IgM (48-271 mg/dL): These antibodies are found in the blood and lymph fluids. They are produced by the body in response to an infection and help the immune system fight it.

- HIGH (protein content): liver and kidney damage, TB, respiratory problems, alcoholism, rheumatoid arthritis, leukemia, and dehydration

- LOW (protein content): liver and kidney malfunction, burns, severe diarrhea, hormonal imbalance, digestive problems, malnutrition

- See Antibody Serum Tests in the Appendix.

IgA (81-463 mg/dL)

Selective deficiency of IgA is the most common immune deficiency disorder. Persons with this disorder have a low or absent level of a blood protein called Immunoglobulin A. IgA deficiency is usually inherited (passed down through families); however, cases of drug-induced IgA deficiency have been reported. IgA's effect on the body focuses on food allergies.

- HIGH: chronic hepatitis, liver disease, rheumatoid arthritis and cancer of plasma cells

- LOW: (symptoms) bronchitis, kidney problems, enteropathy, leukemia, ear infections, sinusitis, lung infections, skin infections, conjunctivitis, drugs, diarrhea, Crohn's disease, colitis, mouth infections

- Complications: Autoimmune disorders such as rheumatoid arthritis, systemic lupus and celiac sprue may develop. Patients with IgA deficiency may develop antibodies to IgA, which can have severe life-threatening reactions to blood transfusions and blood products.

- Note: If transfusion is necessary, washed cells may be cautiously given.

- Ways to improve your results: Balance gut and intestinal flora with probiotics and digestive enzymes.

- See Antibody Serum Tests in the Appendix.

IgE (<115 KU/L)

IgE is the least abundant in the body but has the most powerful effect. IgE mediates allergic reactions, including life-threatening ones called anaphylaxis. IgE reacts with mast cells that contain histamine which induces allergy symptoms (e.g. rash, itching, hives, swollen lymph nodes, runny nose, sneezing).

IgE is found mainly in the lungs, skin and mucous membranes. For people who are allergic to dairy foods, shellfish, peanuts and certain medications, IgE is driving the reaction.

- HIGH: asthma, food allergies, seasonal allergies, rhinitis, parasitic infections, atopic dermatitis, eczema, some autoimmune diseases

- LOW: muscle disease

- Ways to improve results: Monitor for food allergies or intolerances, eat organic, support digestive health, avoid foods known to be high in allergens and take supplements to lower histamine levels.

- Helpful nutrients (to lower histamine): vitamin C, quercetin, probiotics, rutin, homeopathics

- Helpful herbs: butterbur, mangosteen, nettles, licorice, wild oregano

- See Antibody Serum Tests in the Appendix.

IgG (694-1618 mg/dL)

This is the most abundant immune globulin in the body but the smallest in terms of size. They are found throughout the body and make up over 75% of our antibodies. They stay with us all of our lives. They enhance our immune system via increased "phagocytosis" which is the ability of white blood cells to gobble up and neutralize foreign invaders (e.g. toxins, parasites, poisons, heavy metals, viruses, bacteria). IgG antibodies (useful in food allergies) and be tested with the ELISA test.

- HIGH: chronic infections (Epstein-Barr virus), MRSA, Lyme disease, multiple myeloma, psoriasis, MS, systemic lupus, Bartonella bacteria, HIV, hepatitis

- LOW: leukemia, kidney damage, lymphoma, recurrent infections, heredity, prophylactic antibiotic treatment, macroglobulinemia, some forms of nephrotic syndrome

- Ways to improve results: Heal digestive problems with diet or nutrients. Attempt to reduce histamine levels.

- Helpful nutrient: vitamin C, quercetin, bioflavonoids

- Note: See IgE for ways to lower histamine.

- See Antibody Serum Tests in the Appendix.

IgM (48-271 mg/dL)

The IgM is the largest of all immune molecules. It is highly efficient and has 10 different antigen biding sites. IgM is the first responder when you attract an infection (virus and/or bacteria). It is found primarily in lymph.

Patients with Hyper-IgM (HIGM) syndrome are susceptible to recurrent and severe infections and in some types of HIGM syndrome, opportunistic infections and an increased risk of cancer, as well. The disease is characterized by decreased levels of immunoglobulin G (IgG) in the blood and normal or elevated levels of IgM. A number of different genetic defects can cause hyper-IgM.

- HIGH: in the initial phase of a bacterial, viral or fungal infection (sometimes can remain elevated for years), viral hepatitis, kidney damage, MONO, cancer of the lymph cells, nephrotic syndrome, parasites, Lyme disease, various autoimmune diseases

- LOW: multiple myeloma, leukemia, Hashimoto's thyroiditis, anemia, lupus, some inherited immune disorders

- See Antibody Serum Tests in the Appendix.

INR (International Normalization Ratio) (1-2 normal value)

The INR is a standardized way of expressing the PT value. The INR ensures that PT results obtained by different laboratories can be compared. It is important to monitor INR (at least once a month and often twice weekly) to make sure that the level of warfarin remains in the effective range.

- HIGH: increased risk of bleeding. Patients taking warfarin must have their blood tested so frequently.

- LOW: blood clots can occur

- Ways to improve your results (that may lower INR): Consuming beef and pork liver (high in vitamin K) will lower INR levels. Veal, lamb, chicken, turkey and meats have lower levels of vitamin K and can lower INRs.

- Risky nutrients (that can increase INR): grapefruit juice, bitter orange, Cat's claw, chrysin, cranberry, devil's claw, DHEA, echinacea, eucalyptus, feverfew, garlic, goldenseal, ipriflavone, kava, licorice, lime, milk thistle, peppermint, red clover, resveratrol, sulforaphane, valerian, wild cherry

- Note: Be careful consuming these nutrients and herbs when taking blood thinners (e.g. warfarin).

- Complications: If you experience the following signs of bleeding, call 9-1-1 or your healthcare provider immediately: severe headache, confusion, weakness or numbness, coughing up large amounts of bright red blood, vomiting blood, bleeding that will not stop, bright red blood in stool.

Insulin, serum (5-30 mcU/L)

Insulin is the hormone made by the pancreas (although the stomach can secrete small amounts). Serum insulin levels help to evaluate insulin production by the beta cells in the pancreas to help diagnose the presence of an insulin-producing tumor in the islet cells of the pancreas (insulinoma), to help determine the cause of low blood sugar (hypoglycemia), to help identify insulin resistance or to help determine when a type 2 diabetic might need to start taking insulin to supplement oral medications.

For a blood test, you must fast for 12 hours. Your blood insulin will be measured every half hour and should return to normal after 4 hours.

- HIGH: liver disease, pancreatic disease, tumors, abnormally large bones, hypothyroidism
- FALSE HIGH: hormones, post-surgery, obesity
- LOW: diabetes, heart attack, low blood glucose symptoms (e.g., sweating, palpitations, dizziness, fainting)
- FALSE LOW: hormone-suppressors, stress
- Ways to improve your results: Consume a diet geared toward balancing blood sugar (more vegetarian).
- Helpful nutrients (to lower insulin sensitivity): vitamin D, zinc, magnesium, vitamin C, essential oils (e.g., cinnamon, rosemary, geranium, basil, eucalyptus)
- Helpful nutrient (to increase insulin sensitivity): omega-3 fatty acids, green tea, more fiber

Insulin-like Growth Factor (IGF-1) (65-225 ng/ml) (highly dosage-age related)

This insulin-like growth hormone, also called somatomedin C, identifies growth hormone deficiency. In children, it can measure slow growth or short stature. This test can evaluate pituitary function and more recently has been relied upon to optimize current dietary and lifestyle strategies in treating cancer. Always check for pituitary disorder.

IGF-1 hormone helps promote normal bone and tissue growth development. In pituitary testing, IGF-1 can detect a deficiency causing hypopituitarism.

- HIGH: pregnancy, pituitary tumors, cancers (e.g. prostate, colorectal, multiple myeloma, breast, lung, thyroid, bone and ovarian)
- LOW: short stature, delayed development in a child, pituitary dysfunction, trauma, infection, inflammation, anorexia, chronic kidney or liver disease
- FALSE LOW: proton-pump inhibitor drugs, Metformin
- Ways to improve your results (to lower IGF-1): Fasting, caloric restriction, reduce animal protein consumption, reduce whey protein consumption and eat a Mediterranean diet.
- Ways to improve your results (to increase IGF-1): Eat prunes, meat, extra protein, milk and whey proteins and methionine.

Iodine, serum (3.2-6.5 ng/100ml)

Iodine is a chemical element. The body needs iodine but cannot make it; the needed iodine must come from the diet. As a rule, there is very little iodine in food, unless it has been added during processing, which is now the case with salt. Most of the world's iodine is found in the ocean, where it is concentrated by sea life, especially seaweed. Average daily intake: 150 micrograms (mcg) per day for adult men and women; 220 mcg for pregnant women; 290 mcg for lactating/breastfeeding women.

The thyroid gland needs iodine to make hormones. If the thyroid doesn't have enough iodine to do its job, feedback systems in the body cause the thyroid to work harder. This can cause an enlarged thyroid gland (goiter). As a trace mineral, iodine comprises only 0.00004% of the human mineral content.

- HIGH (caution in): pregnancy, auto-immune thyroid disease, thyroid tumor, a type of rash called dermatitis herpetiformic

- LOW: radiation exposure, thyroid conditions, leg ulcers, slow mental reaction, fatigue, hypotension, enlarged goiter, hypothyroidism, slow pulse, low libido

- Note: Use caution as iodine may interfere with the absorption of drugs such as ACE-inhibitors, amiodarone, lithium, thyroid medications and diuretics.

- Ways to improve your results (to raise levels): Iodine is present naturally in soil and seawater. The availability of iodine in foods differs in various regions of the world. Individuals in the United States can maintain adequate iodine in their diet by using iodized table salt (unless you have to restrict the amount of salt in your diet) and by eating foods high in iodine—particularly, dairy products, seafood, meat, some breads and eggs.

- Helpful nutrients (to raise levels): kelp, iodine supplement, Lugol's solution, taking a multivitamin containing iodine

- Helpful nutrients (to lower levels): The most common foods that reduce thyroid hormone production (when consumed in excess, especially if raw) belong to the mustard family of cruciferous vegetables known as brassicas (e.g., kale, maca, broccoli, cabbage, Brussels sprouts) due to their higher-than-usual levels of sulfur-containing compounds.

Iron, serum (50-180 mcg/dL)

Iron (Fe+) is the active component of hemoglobin (which carries oxygen in the blood). Iron is critical for red blood cells and also needed for cellular energy and healthy muscle and organ function.

- HIGH: iron overload can cause joint pain, fatigue, heart problems and weakness
- FALSE HIGH: birth control pills, excessive vitamin C intake
- LOW: anemia, reduced ferritin levels, slow development in children, fatigue, poor cognition
- Ways to improve your results (to raise): Consume higher iron foods like beetroot, dark green leafy vegetables, nuts, legumes, liver, oysters, iron-fortified foods, avoid excess vitamin C intake.
- Ways to improve your results (to lower): Limit iron-raising foods, donate blood, vitamin K and eat cabbage.
- Helpful nutrients (to raise): Frequently used forms of iron in supplements include (e.g., ferrous iron salts, sulfate and gluconate). Vitamin C can aid in the absorption of iron. Infants

taking 100 mg daily can double iron absorption.

Iron Binding Capacity (TIBC) (250-425 mcg/dL)

Total iron binding capacity (TIBC) is a blood test to see if you have too much or too little iron in the blood. This test helps the doctor know how well that protein can carry iron in the blood.

- HIGH: occurs when the body's iron stores are low (e.g., iron deficiency anemia, late pregnancy
- FALSE HIGH/LOW: fluorides, birth control pills, chloramphenicol, adrenocorticotropin hormone (ACTH)
- LOW: low protein, malnutrition, sickle cell anemia, inflammation, liver disease (cirrhosis)
- See Transferrin (TSAT).

Lactic Acid (Lactate) (4.5-19.8 mEq/L)

Lactic acid is mainly produced in muscle cells and red blood cells. It forms when the body breaks down carbohydrates to use for energy during times of low oxygen levels. Times when your body's oxygen level might drop include during intense exercise and when you have an infection or disease. A buildup of lactic acid during a workout can create burning sensations in the muscles that can slow down or halt your athletic activity. For this reason, it may be desirable to reduce lactic acid buildup in the muscles.

- HIGH: can be caused by heart failure, liver disease, lung disease, severe infection that affects the entire body (sepsis), very low levels of oxygen in the blood (hypoxia)

- LOW: not important

- Ways to improve your results (to lower): Decrease or eliminate excess exercise. Stay hydrated, breathe deeply and stretch after your workout.

- Helpful nutrients (to lower): magnesium, omega-3 fatty acids, B-vitamins, protein, creatine, beta-alanine, sodium bicarbonate (baking soda), sodium citrate (lemons), sodium phosphate, homeopathy

Lactic Dehydrogenase (LDH) (105-333 U/L)

The lactate dehydrogenase (LDH) test measures the amount of LDH in the blood. LDH is most often measured to check for tissue damage. The protein LDH is in many body tissues, especially the heart, liver, kidney, muscles, brain, blood cells and lungs. Lactic dehydrogenase is present in almost all body tissues, so the LDH test is used to detect tissue alterations and as an aid in the diagnosis of heart attack (LDH raises 2 to 10 times after a heart attack in 48-72 hours), anemia and liver disease. Newer injury markers are becoming more useful than LDH for heart attack diagnosis.

Different LDH isoenzymes are found in different body tissues. The areas of highest concentration for each type of isoenzyme are:
LDH-1: heart and red blood cells
LDH-2: white blood cells; LDH-3: lungs
LDH-4: kidneys, placenta, and pancreas
LDH-5: liver and skeletal muscle

- HIGH: blood flow deficiency (ischemia), heart attack, hemolytic anemia, mono, liver disease, low blood pressure, muscle injury and weakness, new abnormal tissue formation (usually cancer), pancreatitis, stroke, tissue death, shock
- FALSE HIGH: aspirin, alcohol, procainamide, fluoride
- LOW: not a problem, a good response to cancer
- Ways to improve your results (to lower): Treat with high doses of vitamin C.
- Note: See a qualified practitioner before initiating high doses of vitamin C (oral or IV).
- See Liver/Gall Bladder Individual Function Tests and Pregnancy Serum Tests in the Appendix.

LDL cholesterol (<100 mg/dL)

Some cholesterol comes from the food you eat and some is made by your liver. It can't dissolve in blood, so proteins carry it where it needs to go. These carriers are called "lipoproteins." Lipoproteins are the compounds that allow non-soluble fats to move through the bloodstream. LDL is a microscopic blob that's made up of an outer rim of lipoprotein that surrounds a cholesterol center. Its full name is "low-density lipoprotein." It appears that LDL actually delivers fats to cells. A normal LDL/HDL ratio is 3.2-3.5.

- HIGH: thought to increase the risk of heart disease, pregnancy, high altitudes
- FALSE HIGH: certain drugs such as asthma medications (e.g.,

albuterol, prednisone, steroid inhalers), birth control pills, sedatives

- LOW: not usually a problem but severely low levels may be caused by HIV-AIDS, malnutrition, chronic anemia and hyperthyroidism
- Ways to improve you results (to lower): A healthy diet and exercise can help cut your LDL levels. Consume foods that are lower in saturated fat and dietary cholesterol. Add more fiber to diet, eat nuts and quit smoking, if necessary.
- Helpful nutrients: plant sterols
- See Cardiac Function Tests in the Appendix.

Lead, serum (0-50 mcg/dL)

Lead is a toxic metal that has no place in the human body. Lead poisoning (also called "plumbism") inhibits the production of hemoblobin (which carries oxygen). We take in lead from environmental pollutants, paint, automobile exhaust fumes, water pipes and contaminated water. Lead is especially dangerous for children. A child who swallows large amounts of lead may develop anemia, severe stomachache, muscle weakness and brain damage. Even at low levels, lead can affect a child's mental and physical growth.

- HIGH: kidney problems, anemia, hearing loss, developmental delay or losing earlier skills, growth problems; very high levels may cause vomiting, stumbling, muscle weakness, seizures, coma
- Ways to improve your results: Detoxification methods set up by a qualified practitioner.

- Helpful nutrients: vitamin C, vitamin B6, vitamin B1, calcium, zinc, EDTA, glutathione, N-acetyl cysteine
- Helpful herbs: garlic, spirulina, chlorella, blue-green algae, essential oils for detoxification (e.g., helichrysum, rrosemary, jummiper berry, coriander)

Lipase, serum (22-51 U/L)

Also called pancreatic lipase, this is a digestive enzyme that helps break down fat. High amounts of lipase may be found in the blood when the pancreas is damaged or when the tube leading from the pancreas (pancreatic duct) to the beginning of the small intestine is blocked.

- HIGH: bile duct or intestinal obstruction, kidney and/or liver disease, pancreatic disease, gall bladder inflammation, perforated ulcers in the gut
- FALSE HIGH: narcotics, some diuretics
- LOW: Indicates that the pancreas is not producing enough of the digestive enzyme lipase. Low levels may be found in people with medical conditions such as cystic fibrosis, Crohn's or celiac disease.
- Ways to improve your results (if low): Stimulate lipase activity by eating more raw foods (75% of diet); Drink coconut milk and mineral water, and exercise regularly. Consume more foods rich in enzymes (e.g., sprouts, avocado, papaya, grapes, raw honey, extra virgin olive oil, raw milk and coconut oil).
- Ways to improve your results (if high): See a physician for possible pancreatic disease.

- Helpful nutrients (if low): Take a digestive enzyme with higher mg. of lipase.

Liver, serum

The liver is considered the most metabolically active organ in our bodies. A majority of our biological reactions take place in the liver. It performs vital functions such as filtering chemicals and bio-chemicals, storage of glycogen (energy) and essential compounds, synthesis of proteins and hormones.

Liver enzyme tests, formerly called liver function tests (LFTs), are a group of blood tests that detect inflammation and damage to the liver. They can also check how well the liver is working. Liver enzyme testing includes ALT, AST, alkaline phosphatase; true liver function tests (LFTs) include PT, INR, albumin and bilirubin.

- HIGH ENZYMES: cirrhosis, fatty liver, liver cancer, metastasis, steatosis, cholecystitis (gallstones), autoimmune liver disease, hepatitis, obesity, celiac disease, MONO, exposure to toxins, Wilson's disease
- FALSE HIGH: statin drugs, synthetic penicillin, anti-epileptic drugs, ciprofloxacin, nitrofurantoin, ketoconazole, isoniazid, fluconazole, glipizide, skullcap, shark cartilage, senna, gentian, chaparral
- ABNORMAL PANEL: Lyme disease
- Ways to improve your results: Limit alcohol intake, eat a more raw food/vegetarian diet.
- Helpful nutrients: glutathione, vitamin C, lecithin

(phosphadylcholine), B-complex, amino acids, lecithin, raw liver extract, SAMe

- Helpful herbs: milk thistle, dandelion, panax ginseng, centella asitica, ginger, evening primrose oil, garlic, alfalfa, aloe, essential oils (e.g., geranium, helichrysum, grapefruit, frankincense, myrrh)
- See Liver/Gall Bladder Individual Function Tests in the Appendix.

Lipoprotein-associated Phospholipase (Lp-PLA2) (120-199 ng/mL)

Lp-PLA2 is a relatively new test that is sometimes used to evaluate a person's risk of developing heart disease (CHD) or to help determine the risk of having an ischemic stroke. Lp-PLA2 is an enzyme that appears to play a role in the inflammation of blood vessels and is thought to promote further hardening of the arteries (atherosclerosis). Recent studies have found that Lp-PLA2 is an independent risk marker for cardiovascular disease (CVD). This test may be ordered in individuals who have elevated lipids levels, high blood pressure (hypertension), or metabolic syndrome (pre-diabetes). Although the Lp-PLA2 test may be sometimes used along with the cardiac-CRP test, it is not affected by other conditions that can cause general inflammation (e.g., arthritis, gout, auto-immune disease), other than cardiovascular disease.

- HIGH: cardiovascular disease (CVD), ischemic state, stroke, other cardiac risk markers
- LOW: no significant
- Ways to improve your results: See ways to lower cholesterol and other lipids.

- See Cardiac Function Tests in the Appendix.**Lyme Disease (IgG, IgM, WB-Western Blot Assay)**

Lyme disease is a bacterial infection (Borrelia burgdorferi) you get from the bite of an infected tick. Lyme is a multi-stage disease caused by a spirochete (another disease-causing germ) transmitted by the tick bite (most commonly a deer tick).

The first symptom is usually a rash, which may look like a bull's eye. As the infection spreads, symptoms such as fever, headache, muscle and joint aches, stiffness and fatigue can occur over weeks, months and years. Lyme disease can be hard to diagnose because you may not have noticed a tick bite. Blood tests are notoriously inaccurate giving negative results. While antibiotics and other prescription meds are certainly helpful in treating the tick-borne infections, experts in natural medicine say there's also a place for holistic remedies in treatment and management. IgG and IgM can also be used to test for Dengue fever.

REFERENCE RANGE:

< 0.90: Negative

0.91-1.09: Equivocal

> 1.10: Positive

- HIGHER LAB TEST RESULTS: all inflammatory markets (IL-1, IL-6, CRP, Ferritin, TNF-alpha), liver function tests, coagulation testing

- LOWER LAB TEST RESULTS: platelets, salivary DHEA, cortisol, progesterone and testosterone

- ABNORMAL LAB RESULTS: lipid panel, alkaline phosphatase, thyroid function

- Ways to improve your results: Homeopathy, consume more "green drinks" to provide chlorophyll for better detoxification.
- Helpful nutrients: Lyme may deplete vitamin D, zinc, B-complex. Supplement with a multi-vitamin formula, pancreatic enzymes, vitamin C, vitamin A, vitamin E, selenium and omega-3 fatty acids.
- Helpful herbs: wild oregano, wild curcumin, probiotics, chaga mushrooms, garlic, echinacea, goldenseal, alfalfa, dandelion
- Note: See a qualified practitioner before beginning any treatment protocol.
- See Antibody Serum Tests and Pathogen Serum Test in the Appendix.

Lymphocytes, Absolute (0.7-3.1 10^9 cells/L) (700-3,100 cells/mcL) (20-40%)

Lymphocytes are a type of white blood cell (leukocyte) that is of fundamental importance in the immune system. Lymphocytes are the cells that determine the specificity of the immune response to infectious microorganisms (e.g., virus, bacteria, fungal, parasitic), tumors and other foreign substances. In adults, lymphocytes make up roughly 20 to 40 percent of the total number of white blood cells. They are found in the circulation and also are concentrated in central lymphoid organs and tissues (e.g., spleen, thymus, tonsils and lymph nodes), where the initial immune response is likely to occur. There are three types: B-lymphocytes, T-lymphocytes and natural killer cells.

- HIGH (known as lymphocytosis): acute viral infections (e.g., chicken pox, rubella, cytomegalovirus, Epstein-Barr virus (mono), measles, herpes, certain bacterial infections (e.g., whooping cough), tuberculosis, toxoplasmosis (parasite), colitis, lymphocytic leukemia, lymphoma, stress, chicken pox, neutropenia, Crohn's disease, Addison's disease, hepatitis

- LOW (known as lymphocytopenia): autoimmune disorders (e.g., lupus, rheumatoid arthritis), infections (HIV, viral hepatitis, typhoid fever, influenza), bone marrow damage (chemotherapy, radiation therapy), malnutrition, Hodgkin's lymphoma disease

- FALSE LOW: corticosteroids use, marijuana use, mercury poisoning, food allergies, severe hypothyroidism

- How to improve your results: Consume more high quality protein, limit high fatty foods and drink more water.

- Helpful nutrients (to raise levels): omega-3 fatty acids, quercetin, vitamin C, acidophilus, beta-1,3-glucan, CoQ10, acetyl-L-carnitine, zinc, selenium, vitamin B12, other antioxidants

- Helpful herbs (to raise levels): cat's claw, stinging nettle, curcumin, neem, licorice, ashwagandha, astragalus, essential oils (e.g., cypress, sandalwood, lemon)

Magnesium, serum (1.8-3.0 mg/dL)

Magnesium (Mg+) is a trace mineral needed by our muscles and nervous system. It also helps to move small molecules across cell membranes (especially positive-charged electrolyte balance). It makes up only .05% of human mineral content. Magnesium is the most needed mineral to supplement because it is inherently low in the typical

American diet.

- HIGH (very uncommon): adrenal gland underactivity, dehydration, kidney failure, heart problems, hypothyroidism, Addison's disease
- FALSE HIGH: use of antacids and/or laxatives
- LOW: adrenal gland over-activity, burns, constipation, intestinal mal-absorption, low parathyroid function, diabetes, alcoholism, atherosclerosis, respiratory problems, arthritis, kidney stones
- Ways to improve your results: In addition to supplementing (400-600 mg/day for adults), add good foods sources to your diet, such as kelp, wheat bran, almonds, buckwheat, dulse, tofu, pecans, Brazil nuts, Brewer's yeast and beet greens.
- Helpful nutrients: Magnesium supplementation works well with vitamin C, B-complex, vitamin B6, vitamin E, fats, calcium, phosphorus, potassium and sodium.
- See Adrenal Function Tests in the Appendix.

Manganese, serum (15-50 mcg/L)

Manganese is a trace mineral that resembles iron. It is important in activating enzymes and plays a role in glucose metabolism. It is the least toxic of the trace minerals.

- HIGH: edema, liver disease, lung infection, manganese poisoning (from paint, fertilizer, pesticides, manufacturing of glass and drugs)
- LOW: uncommon, epilepsy

- Ways to improve your results: Good food sources include sea vegetables, whole grains, buckwheat, rice, wheat bran and nuts.
- Helpful nutrients: Manganese works with vitamin C, vitamin E, vitamin B1, calcium and phosphorus.
- Note: Supplement with manganese as recommended by a qualified health practitioner.

Mean Cell Hemoglobin (MCH) (25-33 pg)

MCH is a calculation of the amount of oxygen-carrying hemoglobin (red blood cells). It is calculated by dividing the mass of HgB by volume of red blood cells (RBCs).

- HIGH: associated with an increased level of hemoglobin leading to anemia (macrocytic), caused by insufficient levels of folic acid and vitamin B12 (methylcobalamin)
- LOW: caused by iron-deficiency anemia or hypochromic anemia, vitamin deficiency in conjunction with low mean corpuscular volume (small RBCs)
- Ways to improve your results (to raise): Take a potent multi-vitamin-mineral formula with iron (better than eating excess meat for iron).
- Ways to improve your results (to lower): Give blood, drink more water, eliminate meat from your diet and fix sleep apnea.
- Helpful nutrients (to raise): extra folate and vitamin B12

Mean Corpuscular Hemoglobin Conc. (MCHC) (28-36 G/DL)

MCHC is an abbreviation for mean cell hemoglobin concentration, which is the average concentration of hemoglobin in a given volume of blood. MCHC is a calculated value derived from the measurement of hemoglobin and the hemocrit. (The hemoglobin value is the amount of hemoglobin in a volume of blood while the hematocrit is the ratio of the volume of red cells to the volume of whole blood.) The MCHC is a standard part of the complete blood count.

- HIGH (Hyperchromia): an increased usually not a medical problem; autoimmune hemolytic anemia, burn patients, hereditary, may be seen in newborns
- FALSE HIGH: nutritional deficiency
- LOW (Hypochromia): associated with certain types of iron-deficiency anemia (mycrocytic or hypochromic) resulting in hemoglobin deficiency
- Ways to improve your results: homeopathic remedies
- Helpful nutrients (to raise levels): figs, dates, foods high in vitamin C, pamegrante
- Note: See MCV and MCH.

Mean Corpuscular Hemoglobin (MCV) (80-100 FL)

MCV is a measurement of the average size of your red blood cells (RBCs). It may appear normal or small/larger than normal.

- HIGH: indicates large or macrocytic RBCs (anemia), associated with a specific hereditary anemia, increased serum homocysteine, excess alcohol consumption, high altitude

- LOW: internal bleeding, iron anemia, free radicals, intestinal parasites, heavy metal excess, gluten intolerance in gastrointestinal tract, vitamin B6 depletion
- Ways to improve your results (to increase): Supplement with vitamin B12, vitamin B6 and/or folate as instructed by a qualified practitioner.
- Ways to improve your results (to decrease): Utilize a detoxification program.

Mercury, serum (0-2 mcg/dL)

Mercury is a highly toxic element that can be absorbed through the skin and mucous membranes. Mercury can be ingested (contaminated fish), injected (vaccines), implanted (dental amalgams), and/or inhaled (environmental toxins, industrial pollutants). Blood may be an inefficient way to look for mercury poisoning; since the body can't easily eliminate it, mercury will be stored and accumulate in the kidneys, liver and fat.

- HIGH: mercury poisoning symptoms (e.g., metallic taste, vomiting, difficulty breathing, chronic cough, and/or swollen bleeding gums)
- Ways to improve your results: Some people are very good at detoxifying mercury and other toxins, while others store toxins like a toxic waste dump. Eat less fish prone to high mercury, remove mercury-filled amalgams, avoid thiomersal-containing vaccines, drink water, incorporate juicing into your diet and consider chelation therapy.

- Helpful nutrients: glutathione, selenium, vitamin E, Brewer's yeast, vitamin C (high doses), B-complex, L-methionine, L-cysteine
- Helpful herbs: spirulina, chlorella, barley, kelp, apple pectin, garlic, alfalfa, essential oils (e.g., helichrysum, rosemary, geranium)
- Note: Mercury is often linked to chronic candidiasis.

Monocytes, Absolute (0.1-0.9 109 cells/L) (100-900 cells/mcL) (2-8%)

Monocytes, like other WBCs, originate in the bone marrow and spread through body for only 1 to 3 days. Monocytes are responsible for eating foreign intruders, called "phagocytosis." Monocytes make up only 1-3% of total WBC. They can develop into macrophages that attack both viruses and bacteria.

- HIGH (Monocytosis): chronic infections (viral and fungal infections), tuberculosis, infection within the heart (bacterial endocarditis), stress, collagen vascular diseases (lupus, scleroderma, rheumatoid arthritis, TB, vasculitis), monocytic or myelomonocytic leukemia (acute or chronic), other cancers.
- LOW: bone marrow damage or failure, hairy cell leukemia, severe infection, HIV-AIDS
- FALSE LOW: chemotherapy, steroid use
- Ways to improve your results: Consume a healthier (Mediterranean-based) diet with high quality fats, vegetables, fruits, nuts and essential fatty acids (fish). Minimize your intake of sugar and alcohol.

- Helpful nutrients (to lower levels): antioxidants, potent multi-vitamin-mineral supplement
- Helpful herbs (to modulate levels): curcumin, medical mushrooms, essential oils (e.g., oregano, cinnamon, frankincense, melaleuca, lavender)
- Note: See Lymphocytes.
- See Antibody Serum Tests in the Appendix.

Myelocytes % (0-1%)

A myelocyte is a young cell of the granulocytis series occurring normally in the bone marrow (can be found in circulating blood when caused by certain diseases). These cells appear in the circulating blood only in certain forms of leukemia (myelocytic leukemia) or in an overwhelming infection. Myelodysplastic/myeloproliferative neoplasms are a group of diseases in which the bone marrow makes too many white blood cells.

- Note: See Lymphocytes.

Myeloperoxidase Antibodies, IgG, serum (MPA)

MPA is an enzyme in leukocytes (white blood cells) that is linked to inflammation and cardiovascular disease. An elevated blood level of the enzyme predicts the early risk of myocardial infarction (heart attack). MPA is a blood test that evaluates patients suspected of having immune-mediated vasculitis, especially microscopic polyangiitis (MPA), when used in conjunction with other autoantibody tests. It may be useful to follow treatment response or to monitor disease activity in patients with MPA.

- HIGH: coronary plaque erosion in patients with acute coronary syndrome, fatal heart attacks
- LOW: hereditary, leas intoxication, diabetes, leukemia, Hodgkin's lymphoma, aplastic anemia, cancer drugs
- REFERENCE VALUES (for all ages): <0.4 U (negative); 0.4-0.9 U (equivocal); => 1.0 U (positive)

Myoglobin (0-85 mg/ml)

Myoglobin is a protein in the heart and skeletal muscles. When you exercise, your muscles use up any available oxygen. Myoglobin has oxygen attached to it, which provides extra oxygen for the muscles to keep at a high level of activity for a longer period of time. When muscle is damaged, myoglobin is released into the bloodstream and the kidneys help remove it from the body. In large amounts, myoglobin can damage the kidneys.

- HIGH: heart attack, muscular dystrophy, rhabdomyolysis (severe muscle pain), skeletal muscle inflammation, skeletal muscle ischemia (oxygen deficiency), damage to heart muscle
- LOW: not a normal test, but may imply inflammation and rheumatoid arthritis
- Ways to improve your results: Adding enzyme therapy may lower myoglobin (see LDH). Take magnesium and omega-3 fatty acids. Exercise may increase myoglobin levels.

Neutrophil Count, Absolute (2.0-7.5 109 cells/L) (2,000-7,500 cells/mcL) (40-60%)

Neutrophilic granulocytes are the most abundant of the white blood cells and are the most essential component of the immune system. They respond to bacterial infections and other types of inflammation. The primary cells in pus that are observed in a wound are neutrophils.

- HIGH (neutrophilia): acute bacterial infections, inflammation, tissue death (necrosis) caused by trauma, heart attack, burns, intoxications, chronic myelogenus leukemia, stress, neurosis, AIDS
- LOW (neutropenia): sepsis, autoimmune disorders, reaction to drugs, chemotherapy, immunodeficiency, bone marrow damage, radiation, anaphylactic shock, hormonal disorders, parasites, malaria, hepatitis A
- How to improve your results (to lower levels): Consume a strict vegan diet and supplement with vitamin B12.
- How to improve your results (to raise levels): Consume additional starches, meats and desserts.
- Helpful nutrients: In order to modulate the immune system (low or high) take antioxidants, a potent multi-vitamin and omega-3 fatty acids.
- Helpful herbs (low or high): turmeric (curcumin), medical mushrooms, garlic, echinacea, essential oils (e.g., frankincense, oregano, cinnamon, melaleuca)
- See Antibody Serum Tests in the Appendix.

Nucleotidase (5'-NT) (2-17 U/L)

5-Nucleotidase (5'-NT) is a protein produced by the liver. A test can be done to measure the amount of this protein in your blood. It is used mostly to tell if the high protein level is due to liver damage or skeletal muscle damage.

- HIGH: possible liver dysfunction and/or inflammation, use of liver-damaging drugs, cholestasis (blockage of bile), tumor, hepatitis, ischemia (loss blood flow and oxygen) to liver
- FALSE HIGH/LOW: acetaminophen (Tylenol), halothane, isoniazid, methyldopa, nitrofurantoin
- Ways to improve your results: It is difficult to lower 5'-NT but some experts suggest eating a more organic, vegetarian diet.
- See pH Values in the Appendix.

Osmolality (280-300 mOsom/kg)

Osmolality is a test that measures the concentration of all chemical particles found in the fluid part of whole blood (viscosity). When the blood is too thick or thin, the pituitary sends a hormonal message to the kidney to slow down (or speed up) the excretion of water.

- HIGH: diabetes, high blood sugar levels (hyperglycemia), stroke, dehydration, head trauma
- LOW: adrenal gland imbalance, lung cancer, drinking too much water or dilute fluid, low sodium level, underactive thyroid gland
- Ways to improve your results: Balance your pH (see pH).
- See Complete Metabolic Blood Panel and pH Values in the Appendix.

Oxygen Saturation (SO2) (95-100%)

In medicine, oxygen saturation (SO2) measures the percentage of hemoglobin binding sites in the bloodstream occupied by oxygen. At low partial pressures of oxygen, most hemoglobin is deoxygenated. Oxygen saturation combines the value of blood oxygen content and capacity to indicate how much oxygen is available to the body.

- HIGH: unlikely, although hyper-ventilating (panting) may increase values

- LOW (hypoxemia): asthma, blood disease (excess RBCs), lung disease (COPD) and respiratory impairment

- FALSE LOW: excessive exercise

- Ways to improve your results: Exercise more, drink fresh juices, practice breathing techniques, and consume iron rich foods.

- Helpful nutrients (to raise): add extra vitamin E and vitamin C to quench free radicals (oxidative stress) and balance your pH

Parathyroid (PTH protein) (14-64 PG/ml)

The parathyroid hormone-related protein (PTH-RP) test measures the level of a hormone in the blood, called "parathyroid hormone-related protein." This test is done to find out whether a high blood calcium level is caused by an increase in PTH-related protein. No detectable level of PTH is normal.

- HIGH: caused by low calcium levels. PTH-related protein can be produced by many different kinds of cancers, including lung, breast, head, neck, bladder and ovaries, as well as leukemia

and lymphoma, thirst, nausea, fatigue.
- LOW: sarcoidosis, low magnesium, radiation damage, autoimmune diseases, high calcium, tingling, muscle cramps, abdominal pain
- Ways to improve your results (for hyper-parathyroid): Take extra vitamin D.
- Ways to improve your results (for hypo-parathyroidism): Lower your vitamin D2 and D3 levels as recommended by a qualified practitioner.
- See Thyroid Function Tests in the Appendix.

Partial Pressure of Carbon Dioxide (PCO2), arterial (35-45- mm Hg)

Partial pressure of carbon dioxide (pCo2) reflects the amount of carbon dioxide gas dissolved in the blood. Indirectly, the pCO2 reflects the exchange of this gas and shows how rapidly and deeply the individual is breathing.

- HIGH: pulmonary edema, lung disease
- LOW: hyperventilation, hypoxia, anxiety, pregnancy, pulmonary embolism
- Ways to improve your results: Stimulate respiration. See pH.

Partial Thromboplastin Time (PTT) (<60-70 seconds)

The PTT is used primarily to investigate unexplained bleeding or clotting. It may be ordered along with a prothrombin (PT) test to evaluate hemostasis, the process that the body uses to form blood clots to help stop bleeding. These tests are usually the starting points for investigating excessive bleeding or clotting disorders. Partial PTT is made from platelets and tissues.

- SHORTENED: bile obstruction, liver disease, extensive cancer (e.g., ovarian, colon, pancreatic), except when liver is involved
- FALSE SLOW: anticoagulants (heparin)
- TOO PROLONGED (abnormal): thrombocytopenia, vitamin K deficiency, disseminated intravenous coagulation, Factor XII or Factor XI deficiency, Hemophilia A or B, hypo-fibrinogenemia, malabsorption, infection, excessive bleeding

pH (Potential of hydrogen ions) 7.35-7.45

One of the most important bases of a healthy life is a balanced blood pH, or the number of hydrogen ions in a solution (+ charged, acidic or – charged bicarbonate alkaline). Normally, human blood is slightly alkaline. The consistency of the blood pH is essential to the body's ability to maintain a relatively stable internal environment. In fact, humans cannot live if the blood pH falls below 7.0 or above 8.0

The acid-base balance is a critical factor in the health and functioning of the body. Optimal health depends on the body's ability to maintain a slightly alkaline state. Manipulation of the extracellular and/or intracellular pH of tumors may have considerable potential in cancer therapy. Alkaline therapy may enable tumor-selective release of cytotoxic drugs encased in pH-sensitive nanoparticles.

- HIGH (blood is too alkaline): can cause coma, adrenal overactivity, buildup of carbon dioxide (respiratory hyperventilation), lightheadedness

- LOW (blood is too acidic): can be caused by loss of carbon dioxide (respiratory acidosis), emphysema, lung disease, too much water in blood, overstimulation of nervous system, spasms, convulsions, acid reflux, sore muscles, hypoglycemia, brain fog, constipation

- FACTORS LEADING TO ACIDIC pH: Candida infection, dysbiosis, diet-induced, toxicity from acid-forming compounds, alcohol, dysfunction of lungs, kidneys, skin, liver or gastrointestinal tract, dehydration, chronic deficiency of major electrolytes (e.g., sodium, magnesium, calcium, potassium), lactic acid

- Ways to improve your results: Consume an alkalizing diet to raise pH. Take sodium bicarbonate (baking soda), and supplement mineral electrolytes and pancreatic enzymes.

- Helpful foods: avocado, coconut, flaxseed, olive oil, pomegranate, lemons, limes, ginger, garlic, lentils, quinoa, chia seeds, buckwheat, most nuts (except peanuts), plums, cauliflower, eggplant, snow peas, kale, cabbage, spinach, alfalfa, broccoli, pumpkin, and sea salt

- Acid foods (minimize consumption): soft drinks, jams, jelly, alcohol, energy drinks, cheese, pasta, meats, coffee, beer, chocolate, white flour and wheat, artificial sweeteners, white vinegar, wine, ice cream and sugar.

- See pH Values in the Appendix.

Phenylalanine (1-5 U)

Serum phenylalanine screening is a blood test to look for signs of the disease phenylketonuris (PKU). The test detects abnormally high levels of an amino acid called phenylalanine. This test is done to screen infants for (PKU), a relatively rare condition that occurs when the body lacks a substance needed to breakdown the amino acid phenylalanine.

- LOW: depression, hypothyroidism, learning, hypertension, memory function (mental disorders), poor food-burning oxidation, Parkinson's disease, addiction

- Ways to improve your results: Food sources include pumpkin seeds, bee pollen, lentils, cashews, lima beans, peas and sesame seeds.

- Helpful nutrients: vitamin C, vitamin B6

Phosphorus, serum (2.3-4.7 mg/dL)

Phosphorus is a mineral involved in bone metabolism, stronger teeth, improved nerve function and helps muscles contract. Phosphorus acts in the intestines for pH balance.

- HIGH (Hyperphosphatemia): constipation, bone metastasis, kidney disease, hypo-parathyroidism, meat eaters, diabetic ketoacidosis, heart disease, low calcium levels, bone tumors, fractures, cirrhosis

- FALSE HIGH: anticoagulants, synthetic estrogens, excess vitamin D, steroids, alcohol abuse, overuse of antacids

- LOW: (Hypophosphatemia): diabetic coma, severe malnutrition, septicemia, hyperparathyroidism, diarrhea and vomiting, liver disease, high calcium, prolonged hypothermia, hyperinsulinism in non-diabetic patient, vitamin D deficiency

- FALSE LOW: antacids, glaucoma meds, diabetic drugs, insulin, diuretics
- Ways to improve your results (if high levels): Avoid foods high in phosphorus (e.g., pork, cod, salmon, dairy products, tuna and yogurt).
- Ways to improve your results (if low levels): Eat more of the above high-phosphorus foods. Improve digestion, which can cause poor absorption.
- Helpful nutrients (if low levels): vitamin D3, calcium-phosphorus-magnesium vitamin formula, Phos-food drops
- See Kidney Renal Function Tests and Pregnancy Serum Tests in the Appendix.

Platelets (Thrombocytes) (150-400 thous./mcL)

Platelets are little pieces of blood cells. Platelets help wounds heal and prevent bleeding by forming blood clots. Your bone marrow makes platelets. Problems can result from having too few or too many platelets, or from platelets that do not work properly. The average lifespan of a platelet is 7.5 days.

- HIGH (Thrombocytosis): too many platelets, you may have a higher risk of blood clots, leukemia, renal failure, cancer, iron-deficiency and hemolytic anemia, stroke, heart attack, arthritis, inflammatory conditions, rheumatoid arthritis
- FALSE HIGH: aspirin use, high altitude, strenuous exercise
- LOW (Thrombocytopenia): increased risk for mild to

serious bleeding, bruising, trauma, nosebleeds, anemia, bone marrow suppression, HIV, cirrhosis, gastrointestinal bleeding, heavy menstruation, viral infections, sepsis, Lyme disease, autoimmune disease (e.g., systemic lupus, rheumatoid arthritis), chemotherapy and excess radiation

- FALSE LOW: antibiotics, non-steroidal anti-inflammatory drugs (NSAIDs), deficiency of folic acid and vitamin B12, colchicine, H2-blocking drugs, isoniazid, some diabetic drugs
- Note: This test measures and calculates the average size of platelets. This is also referred to as Mean Platelet Volume (MPV) (7.5-11.5 FL), which calculates the size of platelets.
- Ways to improve your results (to lower): Consume a more macrobiotic diet, less dairy foods, less sugar and more super-greens.
- Helpful nutrients (to lower levels): raw garlic, ginseng, ginkgo, pomegranate, omega-3 fatty acids
- Helpful nutrients (to raise levels): shark liver oil, vitamin K, berberine
- See Liver/Gall Bladder Individual Function Tests in the Appendix.

Porphobilinogen (PBG) (0-0.2 mg/100ml)

Porphobilinogen (PBG) is measured in patients with symptoms that suggest acute intermittent porphyria, variegate porphyria, or hereditary coproporphyria. Individual results should be examined in the context of the reference range provided by the performing laboratory. Normally, they leave your body through urine or stools. Porphyria is a genetic or inherited disorder of certain enzymes that participate in the production of heme, that manifests neurological complications and skin problem is 7.5 days.

- HIGH: hepatitis, lead poisoning, liver cancer, porphyria, hepatic coproporphyria
- FALSE HIGH: aspirin, morphine, chloral hydrate, barbiturates, birth control pills
- Note: See Porphyrins, Hemoglobin.

Porphyrins (16-60 mcg/dL)

Porphyrins are a group of organic compounds that help to form many important substances in the body. One of these is hemoglobin (heme), the protein in red blood cells that carries oxygen in the blood. Three porphyrins can normally be measured in small amounts in human blood: copropor-phyrin, protoporphyrin, uroporphyrin.

Porphyria refers to a group of disorders that result in a build-up of natural chemicals that produce porphyrin in your body. It mainly affects your nervous system, skin and other organs. Porphyria is usually inherited; one or both parents pass along an abnormal gene to their child.

- Coproporphyrin (<2.0 mcg/dL): congenital porphyria, sideroblastic anemia
- Protoporphyrin (16-60 mcg/dL): anemia, congenital protoporphyria, increased erythropoiesis, infection, iron deficiency anemia, lead poisoning
- Uroporhyrin (<2.0 mcg/dL): congenital erythropoietic porphyria
- ACUTE SIGNS: severe abdominal pain, nausea, constipation, seizures, hypertension, peripheral neuropathy (e.g. tingling, numbness, or pain in the hands and feet), muscle weakness and pain, confusion, hallucinations, ADHD, autism, anxiety disorders,

depression, Asperger syndrome; or cutaneous porphyrias, a sensitivity to the sun causing burning pain, itching, fragile skin, blisters, scars, increased hair growth, red or brown urine.

- Ways to improve your results: It is important that persons with acute porphyria avoid crash diets with decreases in daily carbohydrate and caloric intakes. Avoid obesity, take vitamin D and extra amino acids.
- Helpful nutrients: vitamin B6, zinc, gamma-linoleic acid, manganese, B-complex, biotin, wild oregano
- Note: May be associated with Candida overgrowth in combination with leaky gut syndrome.

Potassium, serum (3.0-5.3 mEq/L)

Potassium (K+) is a positively-charged electrolyte mineral found in large amounts in our body. It is responsible for healthy heart and muscle function (heartbeat), nerve impulses and regulates the enzymes responsible for metabolizing starches and sugars. Potassium is abundant in both animal and plant tissue, and makes up 5% of the body's mineral content.

- HIGH (Hyperkalemia): cardiac arrest, heart beat irregularity, death, adrenal cortex deficiency, breathing restrictions, cell damage, metabolic acidosis, muscle damage, paralysis, bradycardia
- FALSE HIGH: potassium-sparing diuretics, ACE inhibitors, immune suppressant drugs, NSAIDs, tobacco smoke
- LOW (Hypokalemia): may weaken the heart, increases stroke risk by 2.6 times, vomiting, imbalance of glucose and/or insulin

utilization, adrenal cortex over activity, cystic fibrosis, starvation
- FALSE LOW: diuretics, anti-hypertensive drugs
- Ways to improve your results (to increase): Consume more bananas, berries, kiwi, avocadoes, greens, lentils, raisons, sardines, spinach and potatoes.
- Ways to improve your results (to lower): Consume healthy low-potassium foods such as carrots, pasta, chicken and apples.
- Helpful nutrients (if low): Oral potassium chloride replacement supplements and magnesium are needed to store potassium in cells.
- Helpful nutrients (if high): baking soda (sodium bicarbonate), calcium, licorice
- See Adrenal Function Tests and Kidney Renal Function Tests in the Appendix.

Pregnenolone, serum (P5) (10-200 mg/dL)

Pregnenolone, or P5, is an endogenous steroid hormone that is known as the mother hormone for the adrenal glands. It is the precursor of the progestogens, mineralocorticoids, glucocorticoids, androgens and estrogens, as well as the neuro-active steroids. Pregnenolone is the precursor (building-block) for all other steroid hormones. It is converted directly into DHEA and/or progesterone.

Pregnenolone keeps brain functioning at peak capacity. It has its highest level in the brain and enhances brain function, repairs brain and nerve tissue, protects cerebral function, and guards against neuronal injury.

- HIGH: pregnancy, adrenal cancer, ovarian cancer, congenital adrenal hyperplasia

- LOW: amenorrhea (no periods), ectopic pregnancy, failure to ovulate, miscarriage, Alzheimer's disease, low mental function, neuronal injury, adrenal stress, autoimmune diseases

- Ways to improve your results (to raise levels): Supplement with bioidentical pregnenolone supplements, raise progesterone levels, avoid foods and herbs that raise estrogen (e.g., black cohosh, dong quai, hops, lavender, licorice, motherwort leaf, rhodiola, red clover blossom, saw palmetto berry, and tea tree oil).

- Helpful nutrients (to raise): vitamin B6, magnesium, zinc, vitamin C, natural progesterone cream, and supplemental pregnenolone under supervision of a qualified practitioner

- See Estrogen Dominance in the Appendix.

Progesterone, serum (2-20 mg/ml)

Serum progesterone is a test to measure the amount of progesterone in the blood. Progesterone is a hormone produced and secreted by the corpus luteum of ovaries right after ovulation to repair the endometrium from implantation of the fertilized egg. Progesterone plays a key role in pregnancy. In response to stress, the brain increases steroid hormone production in the adrenal glands (including cortisol, progesterone, DHEA and testosterone) by releasing ACTH. Progesterone serves as a precursor for cortisol and testosterone. Progesterone, cortisol, DHEA and testosterone then help cool down the stress response.

- HIGH: pregnancy, adrenal cancer, ovarian cancer, congenital adrenal hyperplasia, vaginal dryness, low libido

- LOW: amenorrhea (no periods), ectopic pregnancy, failure to ovulate, poly cystic ovarian syndrome (PCOS), miscarriage, stress/anxiety from adrenal insufficiency
- Ways to improve your results (to raise levels): Use supplemental progesterone (bioidentical) cream as prescribed or formulated by a qualified health professional.
- Helpful herbs (to lower levels): Supplement with natural estrogenic herbs (e.g., chaste berry, dong quai, black cohosh, red clover, ginseng).
- See Estrogen Dominance in the Appendix.

PROGESTERONE IN NORMAL RANGES:

- Male: less than 1 ng/mL
- Postmenopausal: less than 1 ng/mL
- Female (mid-cycle): 5 to 20 ng/mL
- Female (pre-ovulation): less than 1 ng/mL
- Pregnancy 1st trimester: 11.2-90.0 ng/mL
- Pregnancy 2nd trimester: 25.6-89.4 ng/mL
- Pregnancy 3rd trimester: 48-150 to 300 or more ng/mL

Prolactin (2-29 ng/ml); pregnant women (10-209 ng/ml)

Prolactin is a hormone released by the pituitary gland. It stimulates breast development and milk production in women. There is no known normal function for prolactin in men, but it may alter the cells of the prostate gland.

- HIGH (hyperprolactinemia): chest wall trauma, hypothalamic disease, dehydration, hypothyroidism, kidney disease, pituitary tumor, high protein meals, emotional stress.
- LOW: unusual and of no significance
- Ways to improve your results: Consume of a more vegetarian/green-food diet, and homeopathy.
- Helpful nutrients (for men): zinc, vitamin E, vitamin B6
- Helpful herb (for women): chaste tree
- See Pregnancy Serum Tests in the Appendix.

Prostate-specific Antigen (PSA) (below 4 ng/nl)

The PSA test is used primarily to screen for prostate cancer. A PSA test measures the amount of prostate-specific antigen (PSA) in your blood. PSA is a protein produced in the prostate, a small gland that sits below a man's bladder. PSA is mostly found in semen, which also is produced in the prostate. Small amounts of PSA ordinarily circulate in the blood. Men over 60 years of age tend to have slowly increasing levels.

- HIGH: an enlarged prostate (hypertrophy), prostate infection (prostatitis), urinary tract infection, prostate cancer, bladder or prostate biopsy
- LOW: favorable
- Ways to improve your results: Eat a more vegetarian diet,

including tomatoes, pomegranate juice and green tea.

- Helpful nutrients: vitamin B6, zinc, vitamin E, vitamin D3, vitamin C, selenium, essential fatty acids, amino acids, DMG, Co-enzyme Q10
- Helpful herbs: saw palmetto, turmeric, bee pollen, curcumin, soy isoflavones, modified pectin, pygeum, essential oils (e.g., frankincense, helichrysum, fennel, thyme)
- Note: The goal is to lower the pro-carcinogenic from of testosterone called dihydrotestosterone (DHT)
- See Cancer Serum Tests in the Appendix.

Protein, total (6.1-8.1 g/dL)

A total serum protein test measures the total amount of protein in the blood. It also measures the amounts of two major groups of proteins in the blood: albumin and globulin. The body's protein is derived from ingested food and is therefore influenced by the quality of nutrition in your diet. To determine accurate protein levels, these blood tests are utilized: total protein, albumin, globulin, albumin/globulin ratio and fibrinogen.

- HIGH: kidney stress, multiple myeloma, HIV, chronic inflammation, high uric acid
- LOW: bleeding, burns, fatty liver disease, protein malabsorption, malnutrition
- Ways to improve your results (to raise): Avoid excessive use of alcohol. Consume higher quality protein (animal, whey, egg) and plants (hemp, pea, pumpkin, rice).

- Ways to improve your results (to lower): drink more water, eat more complex carbohydrates
- Helpful nutrients: multi-amino acid supplement and DHEA, if thyroid function is low
- See Complete Metabolic Blood Panel and Liver/Gall Bladder Individual Function Tests in the Appendix.

Prothrombin time (PT) (11.0-13.5 seconds)

Prothrombin is a blood protein (sometimes referred to as "factor II") that measures the time it takes for the liquid portion (plasma) of your blood to clot.

- HIGH: Bile duct obstruction, bleeding problems, liver disease.
- FALSE HIGH: vitamin K deficiency
- LOW: antibiotic use, aspirin, sedatives
- Ways to improve your results (to lower): Consume foods higher in vitamin K (e.g., cabbage, meats, broccoli, Brussels sprouts, asparagus, grapes, cayenne pepper, avocadoes, pears, kale, spinach) and use essential oils (e.g., marjoram, coriander).
- See Liver/Gall Bladder Individual Function Tests in the Appendix.

Red Blood Cells (RBCs) (4.2-5.9 cmm)

RBCs are the most common type of blood cells (we have millions).

In every vertebrate organism, red blood cells are the principal means to deliver oxygen to the body's tissues via blood flow. RBCs are rich in hemoglobin (an iron-containing bio-molecule) responsible for red color of blood.

- HIGH (polycythemia): renal disease, cardiovascular disease, pulmonary disease, high altitude, tobacco use, alcoholism, anemia (deficient folate, vitamin B12), dehydration, lung disease, kidney tumor
- FALSE LOW: cigarette smoking
- LOW (anemia): iron-deficiency anemia, systemic lupus, Addison's disease, acute or chronic bleeding, vitamin B12 and/or folic acid deficiency, bone marrow damage, chronic inflammation, kidney failure, Hodgkin's lymphoma
- Ways to improve your results (to raise): Incorporate more iron-rich red foods, such as red beets, roses, yellow dock root and red clover.
- Ways to improve your results (to lower): Supply oxygen, take oxygen-boosting drops.
- Helpful nutrients: boost iron (if low levels) with drug or plant-based iron (with extra vitamin C to aid in iron absorption), a multi-vitamin-formula, raw liver extract, copper (if low), blue green algae, folic acid, vitamin A (retinol), vitamin C

Red Cell Distribution (RDW) (11-15%)

Red cell distribution width (RDW), which may be included in

a CBC (Complete Blood Count), is a calculation of the variation in the size and shape of red blood cells. In this case, "width" refers to the measurement of distribution, not the size of the cells.

- HIGH: Iron deficiency anemia, bone marrow disorder, reticulocytosis, liver disease
- FALSE HIGH: lack of iron, vitamin B12, folate, nutritional deficiency
- LOW: normal, not important
- How to improve your results: Eat a healthy diet encompassing a variety of foods and supplement as directed by a qualified health practitioner.

Renin (0.2-0.4 ng/ml/hr)

Renin is a protein enzyme released by special kidney cells when you have a decreased salt (sodium) level or low blood volume. When blood in the kidneys are decreased, renin causes blood vessels to narrow (thereby allowing more blood flow to the kidneys), which increases blood pressure.

- HIGH: adrenal tumors, blood loss (hemorrhage), hypertension, kidney injury or tumor, dehydration, heart failure
- LOW: hypotension, high salt intake, blood transfusion, steroid drug use
- Ways to improve your results (to lower): Any means from food, prescription or natural medicines that will lower blood pressure.
- Helpful nutrients (to lower): vitamin D3

Resin T3 Uptake (T3RU)

The T3RU test measures the level of proteins that carry thyroid hormone in the blood. This can help your healthcare provider interpret the results of T3 and T4 blood tests. Because the free T4 blood test and TBG blood tests are available, the T3RU test is rarely used now.

- Note: See Thyroid Binding Globulin Hormone.

Retic Count (Reticulocytes) (0.5-2.0%), absolute (20-80,000 cells)

Reticulocytes are immature red blood cells. Retic count is used to determine if the bone marrow is functioning properly and responding adequately to the body's need for red blood cells (RBCs). Also used to help detect and distinguish between different types of anemia.

- HIGH: overproduction of red blood cells leading to bleeding (hemorrhage)
- LOW: iron anemia from deficiency of vitamin B12 and/or folic acid, radiation and chemotherapy, severe kidney disease
- See RBCs.

Reticulocytes (0.5-2.0%)

A reticulocyte count is a blood test that measures the percentage of reticulocytes in the blood. Reticulocytes are slightly immature red blood cells.

- HIGH: hemolytic anemia, pregnancy, bleeding, blood disorder in a fetus or newborn known as erythroblastosis fetalis, kidney disease
- LOW: bone marrow failure (for example, from drug toxicity,

tumor, radiation therapy or infection), cirrhosis, anemia caused by low iron levels, chronic kidney disease, low levels of vitamin B12 or folate

- Ways to improve your results: Support the kidneys via good nutrition.
- Helpful nutrients: vitamin B12, folate and B-complex as recommended by a qualified practitioner

Rheumatoid factor (RF) (positive or negative) (<40-60 U/ml)

Rhesus (Rh) factor is an inherited trait that refers to a specific protein found on the surface of red blood cells. If your blood has the protein, you're Rh positive—the most common Rh factor. If your blood lacks the protein, you're Rh negative. Although Rh factor doesn't affect your health, it can affect pregnancy.

RF is an antibody to one of the body's white blood cells (specifically a B-lymphocyte or immunoglobulin). This is an instance of "autoimmunity." RF is an antibody that is not usually present in the normal healthy individual.

- HIGH (positive): rheumatoid arthritis, mono, lupus, syphilis, heart disease, lung disease, scleroderma, Sjogren's syndrome, parasites, AIDS, hepatitis, influenza, malaria
- LOW-NORMAL no presence of antibodies
- Ways to improve your results: Lower RF factor with an anti-inflammatory (alkaline) diet, including lemons.
- Helpful nutrients: higher doses of Omega-3 fatty acids
- Helpful herbs: green tea, curcumin, boswellia
- See Antibody Serum Tests and Pathogen Serum Test in the

Appendix.

Sedimentation rate (women: 0-20 mm/hr.; men 0-10; child 0-10)

A sedimentation rate (ESR) is common blood test that is used to detect and monitor inflammation in the body. The sedimentation rate is also called the erythrocyte sedimentation rate because it is a measure of the speed that the red blood cells (erythrocytes) in a tube of blood fall to the bottom of the tube, or sediment. Also ESR may screen for infection.

- HIGH: most autoimmune disease (e.g., rheumatoid arthritis, systemic lupus erythematosus, psoriatic arthritis, TB, reactive arthritis, polymyalgia rheumatica), abscesses, cancer, heart attack, kidney disease, tumors, thyroid disease, infections
- LOW: no usually a concern, bacterial infection, sickle-cell disease, liver disease
- Ways to improve your results (to lower): Limit or eliminate red meat, alcohol, hydrogenated fats, refined sugars, white flour and any foods that encourage inflammatory responses.
- Helpful nutrients: omega 3 fatty acids, flaxseed and flaxseed oil
- Helpful herbs: turmeric (curcumin), ginger
- See Pregnancy Serum Tests in the Appendix.

Serotonin, serum (101-283 ng/ml)

Serotonin is a chemical produced by nerve cells. The serum serotonin level is a blood test to measure the amount of serotonin in your body.

This test may be done to diagnose carcinoid syndrome (a rare cancerous tumor). Many patients with carcinoid syndrome have high levels of serotonin in the blood and urine.

- Note: Serotonin from serum is NOT used to diagnose or treat depression or low mood.

- HIGH: carcinoid syndrome (tumors of the small intestine, colon, appendix, and bronchial tubes in the lungs). Carcinoid tumors have few symptoms but some may include abdominal pain, bright red flushing of the skin, diarrhea, and heart palpitations.

- FALSE HIGH: Serotonin reuptake inhibitors (SSRIs, such as Paxil, Prozac, Lexapro) may make symptoms worse by increasing levels of serotonin.

- Ways to improve your results: Foods can greatly influence the brain's behavior. A poor diet, especially junk food, can lead to depression.

- Note: The substance that processes serotonin is the amino acid tryptophan.

- Helpful nutrients: essential fatty acids, L-tyrosine, 5HTP, SAMe, B-complex, taurine, zinc, choline, magnesium, vitamin C, chromium

- Helpful herbs: ginkgo, St John's wort, Siberian ginseng, kava kava, licorice root, essential oils (e.g., frankincense, lemon, lavender, bergamot)

Sex Hormone Binding Globulin (SHBG)

The test for SHBG is primarily ordered in conjunction with other tests to evaluate the status of a man's androgen (male hormone) levels.

With men, the issue of concern is testosterone deficiency, while with women the concern is excess testosterone production. A total testosterone should be taken prior to the SHBG test.

- HIGH: liver disease, hyperthyroidism, eating disorders (anorexia), estrogen use (hormone replacement therapy and oral contraceptives), hypogonadism
- FALSE HIGH: statin drugs, beta blockers, antifungals, hair loss drugs, antidepressants
- LOW: obesity, Polycystic ovarian syndrome (PCOS), hypothyroidism, hirsutism, steroid use, acne, Cushing disease
- Ways to improve your results (to raise): Add magnesium, take a bioidentical testosterone hormone replacement, zinc, soy, reduce sugar, green tea and coffee.
- Ways to improve your results (to lower): boron, fish oil (omega 3 fatty acids), vitamin D.
- Note: See Testosterone.

Sodium, serum (135-146 mEq/L)

Sodium (Na+) is a positively-charged electrolyte mineral that keeps water (the amount of fluid inside and outside the cell). It is also important in muscle contractions and nerve impulses.

- HIGH: May increase blood pressure, chance of heart failure, kidney damage, diabetes, dehydration, coma, Cushing's syndrome.
- FALSE HIGH: high salt diet, low fluid intake, steroids, diuretics,

sweating, pain-relieving medications

- LOW: uncommon, but can occur in alkalinity deficiency (acidosis) and adrenal over-activity, edema, burns, CHF
- FALSE LOW: too little salt intake, vomiting, diarrhea, diuretics
- Ways to improve your results (if low): Consume foods such as butter, clams, bacon, sardines, sea or table salt, milk and tomatoes.
- Ways to improve your results (if high): Vitamin K1, Omega-3-fatty acids with Coenzyme-Q10.
- See Adrenal Function Tests and Kidney Renal Function Tests in the Appendix.

Sodium Bicarbonate (22-28 mEq/L) HCO3

A bicarbonate ion is a negatively charged electrolyte needed to regulate the acidity of the blood (pH). In the lungs, bicarbonate ions return to gaseous form (carbon dioxide) to be exhaled. Excess secreted through kidneys. In the body, most of the CO2 is in the form of a substance called bicarbonate (HCO3-). Therefore, the CO2 (carbon dioxide) blood test is really a measure of your blood bicarbonate level. Generally, Co2 test is ordered when lung function is being evaluated, and bicarbonate when kidney function is being evaluated. Excess secreted through kidneys.

In the body, most of the CO2 is in the form of a substance called bicarbonate (HCO3-); therefore, the CO2 (carbon dioxide) blood test is really a measure of your blood bicarbonate level. Generally, a Co2 test is ordered when lung function is being evaluated, and bicarbonate when kidney function is being evaluated.

- HIGH: adrenal gland stress, asthma, blood too alkaline, breathing problems, drug overdose, heart disease, starvation
- FALSE HIGH: steroids, diuretics, sweating
- LOW: alcohol and aspirin poisoning, diabetes, diarrhea, fever, hyperventilation, shock, kidney/liver disease, alkalinity deficiency (acidosis adrenal gland stress, asthma
- Ways to improve your results (if low): Take one level teaspoon of (organic) sodium bicarbonate powder in 2-4 ounces of warm or hot water (add lemon to improve taste).
- Ways to improve your results (if high): Consume acidic foods and beverages.
- See Complete Metabolic Blood Panel and Pregnancy Serum Tests in the Appendix.

Testosterone, serum (male: 300 -1,000 ng/dL; (female: 15 – 70 ng/dL)

A testosterone test measures the amount of the male hormone, testosterone, in the blood. Both men and women produce this hormone. The test measures the total amount of testosterone, an anabolic hormone, in the blood. Much of the testosterone in the blood is bound to a protein called "sex hormone binding globulin" (SHBG). Another blood test can measure the "free" testosterone.

- HIGH: resistance to the action on male hormones (androgen resistance), tumor of the ovaries, cancer of the testes, congenital adrenal hyperplasia.
- Note: It is known that elevated dihydrotestosterone (DHT) levels

are pro-carcinogenic (prostate cancer).

- LOW (men): early or late puberty (in boys), infertility, erectile dysfunction, low level of sexual interest, infertility, thinning of the bone, male-pattern baldness or hair thinning, insulin resistance, metabolic syndrome, diabetes, heart disease, osteoporosis, low muscle mass, poor concentration, fatigue, infertility

- Note: It is known that men who undergo greater stress and tension (causing higher cortisol levels) directly suppress testicular production of testosterone.

- LOW (women): acne, oily skin, change in voice, decreased breast size, excess hair growth (thick, dark hair in the area of the moustache, beard, sideburns, chest), irregular or absent menstrual periods, infertility

- Ways to improve your results: Exercise, reduce stress (balance cortisol) and address metabolic syndrome.

- Helpful nutrients (in men): DHEA, zinc, selenium, vitamin D, vitamin B6, L-arginine, nitric oxide

- Helpful herbs (in men): saw palmetto, tribulus, ashwagandha, yohimbe, ginseng, rhodiola

- Helpful nutrients (in women): indole-3-carbonol is a natural supplement made from cauliflower and broccoli, and is known to reduce androgens.

- Helpful herbs (in women): saw palmetto, chaste tree, black cohosh

- See Adrenal Function Tests in the Appendix.

Thyroglobulin Antibodies (<OR=1 IU/ml)

Antithyroglobulin antibody is a test to measure antibodies to a protein called thyroglobulin, which is found in thyroid cells.

- HIGH: Graves' disease, Hashimoto's thyroiditis, hypothyroidism, systemic lupus (SLE), type 1 diabetes, thyrotoxicosis
- Note: See Thyroxine, serum.
- See Thyroid Fuction Tests in the Appendix.

Thyroid Peroxidase (TPO) antibodies (<9 IU/ml)

Thyroid antibody testing is primarily ordered to help diagnose an autoimmune thyroid disease (e.g., Hashimoto's disease, Graves' disease, cancer) and to distinguish it from other forms of thyroid dysfunction. It may be ordered to help identify a goiter or other signs and symptoms associated with high or low thyroid hormone levels and as a follow-up to normal TSH, T3 or T4 testing.

- HIGH: Elevated TPO levels are found in virtually all cases of Hashimoto's disease and they will also be raised in 65% of patients with Graves' disease.
- Ways to improve your results: Eat a gluten-free, organic diet.
- Helpful nutrients: selenium (Brazil nuts), vitamin C, vitamin D, iodine, progesterone (see a qualified practitioner).
- See Thyroid Function Tests in the Appendix.

Thyroid Stimulating Hormone (TSH) (0.40-4.50 mIU/L)

TSH is the hormone that controls the thyroid gland. An excess or deficiency of TSH can affect energy levels, mood and many other functions. When the thyroid gland begins to fail, due to primary disease, TSH levels increase. This condition is called primary hypothyroidism, or low function of the thyroid gland.

If TSH levels decrease, the gland is overactive and produces too much thyroid hormone. This is called primary hyperthyroidism. Thus, TSH helps distinguish a sick person (with thyroid problems) from a sick person (without thyroid problems).

- HIGH (hypothyroidism): Graves' disease, toxic nodular goiter, excess iodine levels in gland, TSH antibodies, Hashimoto's thyroiditis
- FALSE HIGH: prednisone, lithium, amiodarone, dopamine, iodide
- LOW (hyperthyroidism): overactive gland, excess amount of thyroid hormone medication, damage to pituitary gland
- FALSE LOW: dopamine, glucocorticoids
- Ways to improve your results (to lower): Treat underlying conditions like food allergies, gluten, heavy metals, nutritional deficiencies, and exercise and minimize stress.
- Ways to improve your results (to raise): Exercise and optimize nutrition (avoid excess soy and isoflavones).
- Helpful nutrients (to lower): zinc, selenium, foods that contain iodine, zinc, omega-3 fatty acids, essential oils (e.g., peppermint, clove)

- Helpful herbs (to raise): motherwort, bugleweed, lemon balm, broccoli, essential oils (e.g., myrrh, lemongrass)
- Note: See qualified health practitioner regarding TSH balancing.
- See Thyroid Function Tests in the Appendix.

TSH LEVELS (these references are only applicable to pregnant females):

- First Trimester: 0.26-2.66 mIU/L
- Second Trimester: 0.55-2.73 mIU/L
- Third Trimester: 0.43-2.91 mIU/L

Thyroid Symptoms (Hypothyroidism)

- Symptoms of hypothyroidism may include:
- Easy weight gain
- Dry and/or puffy skin
- Constipation
- Cold intolerance
- Hair loss, fatigue
- Menstrual irregularity in women
- Enlarged thyroid gland (goiter)
- Ways to improve your results: To test yourself for an underactive thyroid, place a thermometer under your arm for 15 minutes for 5 days. A temperature lower than 97.6 degree F may indicate an underactive thyroid gland.
- Helpful nutrients: kelp, L-tyrosine, raw glandular extract,

B-complex, vitamin B2, vitamin B12, Brewer's yeast, selenium, vitamin C, zinc

- See Thyroid Function Tests in the Appendix.

Thyroid Symptoms (Hyperthyroidism)

- Increased heart rate
- Anxiety, difficulty sleeping
- Weight loss, occasional diarrhea
- Tremors in the hands
- Weakness
- Light sensitivity, visual disturbances
- The eyes may be affected (e.g., puffiness around the eyes, dryness and, in some cases, bulging of the eyes)
- Ways to improve your results: Eat these foods to help suppress thyroid hormone production: broccoli, Brussels sprouts, cabbage, cauliflower, kale, mustard greens. Avoid excessive dairy, soft drinks and nicotine.
- Helpful nutrients: multi-vitamin-mineral formula, B-complex, extra vitamin B1, B2, B6, Brewer's yeast, vitamin C, essential fatty acids
- See Thyroid Function Tests in the Appendix.

Thyroxine-Binding Globulin (TBG) (1.3-2.0 mg/100ml)

The TBG blood test measures the level of a protein that moves thyroid hormone throughout your body. TBG is non-harmful and may be inherited or acquired.

- HIGH: acute porphyria, hypothyroidism, pregnancy (TBG levels are normally increased during pregnancy)
- FALSE HIGH: estrogens, birth control pills, heroin, methadone, phenothiazines
- LOW: hyperthyroidism, malnutrition, nephrotic syndrome, chronic renal failure, liver disease, HIV/AIDS, systemic illness, Cushing syndrome
- FALSE LOW: Depakote, Dilantin, aspirin (high doses), androgens, testosterone, prednisone
- Ways to improve your results: See TSH.
- See Thyroid Function Tests in the Appendix.

Thyroxine, serum (Total T4) (5-13.5 mcg/dL)

Free thyroxine (free T4) tests are used to help evaluate thyroid function and diagnose thyroid diseases, including hyperthyroidism and hypothyroidism, usually after discovering that the TSH level is abnormal. T4 is converted to T3 hormones by the body naturally, but sometimes the body is unable to make this conversion. When your body does not covet T4 to T3, you could become deficient in thyroid hormones.

- HIGH: hyperthyroidism, neonates, acute thyroiditis, hepatitis, liver disease
- FALSE HIGH: birth control pills, heroin, methadone, pregnancy, tamoxifen

- LOW: hypothyroidism or mild sub-clinical hypothyroidism, rare pituitary (secondary) hypothyroidism, low protein intake
- FALSE LOW: aspirin, steroids, drugs for epilepsy, aging, excess protein, sucralfate
- Ways to improve your results (to treat low levels): Consume more foods with high vitamin B and iron, such as fresh vegetables and fruits high in antioxidants, such as cherries, blueberries, tomatoes, squash and peppers.
- Helpful nutrients: zinc, selenium, vitamin D, B-complex, iodine (when needed)
- Note: See T3 and TSH.
- See Thyroid Function Tests in the Appendix.

Thyroxine (Free T4) (0.7-2.0 MG/dL)

Free thyroxine (free T4) tests are used to help evaluate thyroid function and diagnose thyroid diseases, including hyperthyroidism and hypothyroidism, usually after discovering that the thyroid stimulating hormone (TSH) level is abnormal. If severe illness occurs, fT4 may decrease, but it is not a thyroid disease.

- Note: See TSH and T4, serum.
- See Thyroid Function Tests in the Appendix

TORCH

TORCH refers to TOxoplasmosis Rubella Cytomegalovirus Herpes

I and II tests. TORCH is a group of tests run on pregnant women (or sometimes newborns) to determine the child's immunity to viral diseases. The test may be ordered on the newborn when the infant shows any signs suggestive of deafness, mental retardation, seizures, heart defects, cataracts, or enlarged liver or spleen.

- NORMAL: positive in each of 5 tests
- ABNORMAL: negative (lacking immunity)

Total Iron-binding Capacity (TIBC) (250-390 mcg/dL)

Also called Serum Transferrin, total iron-binding capacity (TIBC) is most frequently used along with a serum iron test to evaluate people suspected of having either iron deficiency or overload. These two tests are used to calculate the transferrin saturation, a more useful indicator of iron status than just iron or TIBC alone.

- HIGH: iron deficiency anemia, acute or chronic blood loss, acute hepatitis, late stage pregnancy, chronic illness
- LOW: hemochromatosis, hypoproteinemia, liver cirrhosis, non-iron anemia, infectious disease, iron overload, kidney/ liver disease, hemolytic anemia, malnutrition
- Ways to improve your results (to raise levels): Supplement with hemevite iron and take digestive enzymes.
- Note: See ferritin, HCT, HgB.

Transferrin Saturation (TSAT) (males 15-50%; females 12-45%)

TSAT (measured as a percentage) is a medical laboratory value. It is the ratio of serum iron and total iron-binding capacity, multiplied by 100. The value of the amount of transferrin that is available to bind iron tells a clinician how much serum iron is actually bound. For instance, a value of 15% means that 15% of iron-binding sites of transferrin are being occupied by iron.

- HIGH: iron-deficiency anemia, estrogen therapy, pregnancy
- LOW: chronic infections, renal disease, protein deficiency, acquired liver disease, malnutrition, genetic deficiency, heredity, iron-overload
- Note: See TIBC.

Triiodothyronine, serum (Total T3) (80-220 ng/dL)

T3 is one of the 2 hormones containing iodine produced by the thyroid gland. T3 helps to regulate metabolism (how nutrients are broken down, distributed and utilized) by increasing the rate of chemical reactions. T3-uptake measures how much T3 is attached to its carrier protein in the blood, thus it measures the level of "free" (unbound) hormone.

- See Thyroid Function Tests in the Appendix.

T3 (Free T3) (2.3-4.2 PG/ml) (27-37%)

A free T3 may be ordered when someone has an abnormal TSH test result. It may be ordered as part of the investigative workup when a person has symptoms suggesting hypertension, especially if the free T4 level is not elevated. It is the best marker for measuring the amount of thyroid hormone available for the thyroid receptor sites.

- HIGH/LOW: same as T4
- FALSE HIGH: various prescription drugs, heparin, steroids, aspirin
- See Thyroid Function Tests in the Appendix.

T3, Reverse (rT3) (8-25 ng/dL)

This test measures the amount of reverse T3 that is produced. The production of rT3 usually takes place in cases of chronic or extreme stress, trauma and surgery. It appears that the increased production of rT3 is due to the body's inability to clear rT3, as well as elevated cortisol.

- Note: See cortisol, T3, free T3.
- See Thyroid Function Tests in the Appendix.

Triglycerides (50-150 mg/dL)

Triglycerides are the chemical form in which most fat exists in food and the body. These fats are composed of fatty acids and glycerol. Triglycerides combine with proteins (as a lipoprotein) that transport fats through the bloodstream.

The two main sources of triglycerides are the diet and the liver. Dietary triglycerides are absorbed in the small intestines and secreted into the lymph. The liver also produces triglycerides from fat and carbohydrates. Liver triglycerides are packed with very low-density lipoproteins (VLDL) and secreted in to the blood for the production of receptor sites.

- HIGH: linked to higher coronary artery disease or event; a disorder of fat metabolism from autoimmune disease, alcoholism, diabetes, obesity, kidney-liver disease, pancreatitis, hypothyroidism
- LOW: diets not containing enough fat or inability to absorb fats (possible hyperthyroidism), decreased food intake, increased inflammation, cachexia (body wasting), liver congestion, chronic heart failure
- Ways to improve your results (to lower): Better balance your blood sugar by consuming less refined carbohydrates and saturated fats.
- Helpful nutrients (to lower): omega-3 fatty acids, niacin, pantethine, B-complex, alpha-lipoic acid
- Helpful herb (to lower): turmeric (curcumin), green tea extract, guggulipids
- See Cardiac Function Tests and Complete Metabolic Blood Panel in the Appendix.

Troponin I (0.01-0.03 ng/ml)

A troponin test measures the levels of troponin T or troponin I proteins in the blood. These proteins are released when the heart muscle has been damaged, such as what occurs with a heart attack. The more damage there is to the heart, the greater the amount of troponin T and I there will be in the blood. Even a slight increase in the troponin level will often imply there has been some damage to the heart. Very high levels of troponin are a sign that a heart attack has occurred. Most patients who have had a heart attack have increased troponin levels within 6 hours. After 12 hours, almost everyone who has had a heart attack will have raised levels. Troponin levels may remain high for 1 or 2 weeks after a heart attack.

- HIGH: heart attack, cardiomyopathy, pulmonary hypertension, very rapid heartbeat, coronary artery spasm, congestive heart failure, open heart surgery, myocardial infarction (MI)
- LOW or NORMAL: desirable
- How to improve your results: Avoid strenuous exercise. lower your cortisol (stress) levels, improve kidney function and lower lipids via diet and supplements.

Uric Acid (3.5-7.2 mg/dL)

Uric acid is the end waste product of cell breakdown and purine degradation. Purines are found in some foods and drinks. These include liver, anchovies, mackerel, dried beans, peas and beer. Most uric acid dissolves in blood and travels to the kidneys. From there, it passes out in urine. If your body produces too much uric acid or doesn't remove enough if it, you can get sick.

- HIGH (Hyperuricemia): gout, gouty arthritis, hypertension, arthritis, diabetes, acidosis, high RBCs, cancer, leukemia, liver or kidney damage, kidney stones (10% uric acid), lead poisoning, Down's syndrome, psoriasis, metabolic acidosis, alcoholism
- FALSE HIGH: alcohol, chemotherapy, aspirin, L-dopa, diuretics
- LOW: low zinc levels, kidney disease, Wilson's disease, multiple sclerosis
- Ways to improve your results (to lower): Decrease the consumption of high purine foods (animal protein) and eat a more

plant-based diet.
- Helpful nutrients (to lower): vitamin C, cherries, omega-3 fatty acids, krill oil, B complex, pancreatic enzymes
- Helpful herbs (to lower): boswellia, curcumin, cat's claw, celery seed, apple cider vinegar
- See Complete Metabolic Blood Panel and Kidney Renal Function Tests in the Appendix.

Viral Hepatitis (tests include ALT, AST, Liver panel)

Many illnesses and conditions can cause inflammation of the liver (hepatitis), but certain viruses cause about half of all hepatitis in people. Viruses that primarily attack the liver are called hepatitis viruses. There are several types of hepatitis viruses including types A, B, C, D, E and possibly G. Types A, B, and C are the most common.

All hepatitis viruses can cause acute hepatitis. Some can cause chronic hepatitis, mono (look for cytomegalovirus). Symptoms of acute viral hepatitis include fatigue, flu-like symptoms, dark urine, light-colored stools and jaundice; however, acute viral hepatitis may occur with minimal symptoms that go unrecognized. Rarely, acute viral hepatitis causes hepatic failure.

- Ways to improve your results: Lessen intake of fats, avoid greasy foods, eat brown rice, oatmeal, organic fruits, sea vegetables, wheatgrass, chlorella, buckwheat.
- Helpful nutrients: vitamin A carotenoids, thymus gland extract, vitamin B5, vitamin B12, vitamin C, beta-glucan, ozone, magnesium, CoQ10, DHEA

- Helpful herbs: milk thistle, bitter melon, royal jelly, olive leaf extract, mushrooms, essential oils (e.g., myrrh, melaleuca, frankincense)
- See Antibody Serum Tests in the Appendix.

Vitamin A, serum (50-200 mcg/dL)

The vitamin A test measures the level of vitamin A in the blood

- HIGH: acute toxicity (liver), dry skin, vomiting, alopecia, bone demineralization and pain, hypercalcemia, lymph node enlargement
- LOW: bone or teeth problems in young children, dry or inflamed eyes, hair loss, loss of appetite, night blindness, recurring infections, skin rashes, pancreas problems (pancreatitis), celiac disease, cystic fibrosis
- Ways to improve your results: Supplement with beta-carotene or the synthetic vitamin A (retinol).
- Helpful nutrients: consume more foods high in vitamin A (e.g., carrots, bell peppers, sweet potatoes, dark leafy greens, lettuce, fish, tropical fruits, winter squashes)

Vitamin B12 (400-1100 pg/ml)

A complex organic substance not produced by the body, but is essential for health, particularly the proper formation of RBCs and tissues.

- HIGH: uncommon, possibly blood disease, leukemia, liver disease, excess supplementation

- FALSE HIGH: too much vitamin B12 in diet

- LOW: anemia, pernicious anemia, overactive thyroid, poor diet, intestinal mal-absorption

- FALSE LOW: stomach surgery, pregnancy

- Ways to improve your results (if low levels): Supplement with vitamin B12 tabs or sublingual tabs (1,000-9,000 mcg daily or as directed by a qualified practitioner).

- Helpful nutrients: salmon, mackerel, fortified cereals, milk, liver, sardines

- Note: Ask your physician for vitamin B12 injections sub-cut (methyl form is the best absorbed).

Vitamin C, serum (0.4-1.5 mg/100ml)

Humans do not make their own vitamin C, but we must get this vitamin from food and other sources. Good sources of vitamin C are fresh fruits and vegetables, especially citrus fruits.

- HIGH: diarrhea, possibly formation of vitamin C kidney stones

- LOW: poor iron absorption, age-related vision loss, atherosclerosis, common cold, kidney disease, gall bladder disease, anemia, higher blood pressure, lead poison

- LOW (conditions in which IV vitamin C may be effective): strengthen heart and blood vessels. preventing clots in veins and arteries (atherosclerosis), Lyme disease, hypertension, glaucoma, preventing cataracts, preventing gallbladder disease, preventing dental cavities, constipation, boosting the immune system, hay fever, asthma, bronchitis, collagen disorders, cancer, arthritis and bursitis

- Note: See a licensed practitioner for IV vitamin C treatments.
- Helpful nutrients: camu-camu fruit, berries, kiwifruit, orange peels, dark leafy greens, papaya, broccoli, citrus fruits

Vitamin D, 25-OH, total (30-100 ng/ml)

The 25-hydroxy vitamin D test is the most accurate way to measure how much vitamin D is in your body. In the kidney, 25-hydroxy vitamin D changes into an active form of the vitamin. The active form of vitamin D helps control calcium and phosphate levels in the body.

Vitamin D3 is the potent form of vitamin D called cholecalciferol. Vitamin D, 25-OH, D3 indicates both endogenous production and supplementation. Vitamin D2 (ergocalciferol) is from foods.

- HIGH (Hypervitaminosis D): may be due to excess vitamin D supplementation
- LOW: lack of exposure to sunlight, lack of enough vitamin D in the diet, liver and kidney diseases, poor food absorption, cancer, use of certain medicines, including phenytoin, phenobarbital, and rifampin
- Ways to improve your results: Sunbathe for 15-20 minutes daily when possible or supplement with extra vitamin D3.
- Helpful nutrients (for better absorption): magnesium, calcium vitamin C, vitamin K
- Dietary nutrients: fatty fish (e.g., tuna, salmon, and mackerel),

beef liver, cheese, egg yolks, mushrooms, cow's milk (fortified with 400 IU vitamin D per quart in the USA), cod liver oil

Total 25-HydroxyvitaminD and D3 (25-OH-Vit D):

- <10 ng/mL (critically deficiency)
- 10-19 ng/mL (severely deficiency)
- 20-50 ng/mL (deficient levels)
- 51-80 ng/mL (ideal range)
- 80-100 ng/mL (high but safe)
- >100 (possible complications, toxicity)

VLDL (5-40 mg/dL)

VLDL (very low density lipoprotein) transports cholesterol and triglycerides within the body to fat deposits. It is made in the liver in response to a high-carbohydrate meal. Liver triglycerides are packed with very low-density lipoproteins (VLDL) and secreted in to the blood for the production of energy. Hense, VLDL are lipoprotein particles formed to transport endogenous derived triglycerides to tissues. There is no simple way to calculate VLDL. Some lab results do not give this number. To calculate VLDL: take your total cholesterol and subtract both the HDL and LDL (a good estimate).

- HIGH: conditions known to increase levels include diabetes, obesity and acute hepatitis. It is thought to play a role in atherosclerosis.
- LOW: a healthy response
- Ways to improve your results (to reduce levels): Lifestyle changes

and medications are often successful. Lose excessive weight, avoid s sugary foods and alcohol, exercise and lower triglyceride levels.

- Note: See Total Cholesterol, Triglycerides.
- See Cardiac Function Tests in the Appendix.

White Blood Cells (WBCs) (3.4-10.8 109 cells/L) (3,400-10,800 uL)

WBCs (or leukocytes) play an important role in the health of the immune system. They are produced in the bone marrow and act as the body's protectors against infectious disease and foreign invaders that lead to illness and/or injury. Slightly low WBCs may be a natural level for some people.

When a person gets an infection, WBCs will increase in numbers in order to attack the invader(s). To bring WBC levels back to normal, the spleen and the rest of the lymphatic system (which produces white blood cells, or corpuscles) needs to be brought back to balance.

- HIGH (Leukocytosis): bacterial infections, blood disorders, leukemia, allergies, asthma, tissue damage, anxiety, strenuous exercise, severe stress, inflammation
- LOW (Leukopenia): may be caused by bone marrow disease, most autoimmune diseases, fungal infections, sepsis, lymphoma, anemia, diabetes, viral infections, toxic blood
- FALSE LOW: marijuana
- Ways to improve your results (too raise levels): Anything to build and strengthen the immune system, such as exercise, consuming "green drinks", alkalizing your pH, eating organic yogurt.

- Helpful nutrients (to raise levels): selenium, additional antioxidants, zinc, folic acid, vitamin C, amino acids, CoQ10, acidophilus, lecithin
- Helpful nutrients (to lower levels): grapes, olive oil, soy protein, vinegar, black tea, omega-3 fatty acids, nuts
- Helpful herbs (to raise levels): medical mushrooms, larch bark, Siberian ginseng, astragalus, ashwagandha, echinacea, beta glucan, cat's claw, essential oils (e.g., frankincense, sandalwood, cypress, lemon)
- See Pregnancy Serum Tests in the Appendix.

White Blood Cell Differential Count

The white blood cell differential is often used as part of a complete blood count (CBC) as a general health check. It may be used to help diagnose the cause of a high or low white blood cell (WBC) count, as determined with a CBC. It may also be used to help diagnose and/or monitor other diseases and conditions that affect one or more different types of WBCs. The five types include neutrophils, lymphocytes, monocytes, eosinophils and basophils. The differential totals the number of each type and determines if the cells are present in normal proportion to one another, if one cell type is increased or decreased, or if immature cells are present.

Zinc, serum (0.61-1.10 mcg/ml)

Zinc is a metal. It is called an "essential trace element" because very small amounts of zinc are necessary for human health. Zinc is used for treatment and prevention of zinc deficiency and its consequences, including stunted growth and acute diarrhea in children, and slow wound healing. It is also used for boosting the immune system, treating the common cold.

- HIGH: not common

- LOW: decreased alertness, fatigue, muscle weakness, anemia, prostate problems, lower visual acuity, lower immunity, white specks on fingernails, osteoporosis, ulcers

- Ways to improve your results (to raise levels): Good food sources include wheat germ, oatmeal, sesame flour, pumpkin, squash, pea, lentils and cashews. Lower consumption of foods high in copper (e.g., oysters, sesame seeds, liver, cocoa, seafood).

- Note: Copper and zinc are antithetical in the body. To raise zinc levels, lower copper levels, and vice-versa.

- Note: See a qualified practitioner about supplemental dose, if needed.

APPENDIX

Adrenal Function Tests

- Aldosterone
- Androgens
- Chloride
- Cortisol
- DHEA
- Estrogens (estrone, estriol, estradiol)
- Magnesium
- Potassium
- Sodium
- Adrenal hypofunction: decreased sodium, chloride & glucose; increase potassium
- Adrenal hyperfunction: opposite of above

Antibody Serum Tests

- AIDS/HIV
- Allergies
- ANA
- Bacterial infections
- Blood type
- Hepatitis
- Lyme disease
- Mumps/measles
- Momonucleosis
- Parasites
- Pneumonia
- Rh Factor
- Syphilis
- Toxic shock syndrome
- Toxoplasmosis
- Viral infections

Cardio Function Tests

- C-reactive protein
- Cholesterol, total
- GGTP
- Glucose
- HDL cholesterol
- HDL/LDL ratio
- LDL cholesterol
- Lipid panel
- SGOT (AST)
- SGPT (ALT)
- Triglycerides
- VLDL

Complete Metabolic Blood Panel (CMP)

- Alkaline phosphatase
- Bicarbonate
- Bilirubin
- BUN
- Calcium
- Cardon dioxide
- Glucose
- Osmolality
- pH
- Protein, total
- SGOT (AST)
- SGPT (ALT)
- Triglycerides
- Uric acid

Normal Serum DHEA Levels

- Ages 18-19: 145-395 ug/dL (micrograms per deciliter)
- Ages 20-29: 65-380 ug/dL
- Ages 30-39: 45-270 ug/dL
- Ages 40-49: 32-240 ug/dL
- Ages 50-59: 26-200 ug/dL
- Ages 60-69: 13-130 ug/dL
- Ages >69: 17-90 ug/dL
- Ages 18-19: 108-441 ug/dL
- Ages 20-29: 280-640 ug/dL
- Ages 30-39: 120-520 ug/dL
- Ages 40-49: 95-530 ug/dL
- Ages 50-59: 70-310 ug/dL
- Ages 60-69: 42-290 ug/dL
- Ages >69: 28-175 ug/dL

Estrogen Dominance-Ways to Lower

- Avoid Parabens
- Avoid Bisphenol-A
- Avoid GMO soy
- Avoid over-exposure to chemicals/toxins
- Avoid pesticides and herbicides
- Balance gut flora
- Consume citrus fruits
- Don't use plastic
- Eat cruciferous vegetables
- Eat more organic foods
- Lose weight (body fat stores toxins)

Kidney (Renal) Function Tests

- Albumin
- Blood Urea Nitrogen
- BUN/Creatinine Ratio
- Calcium
- Chloride
- Creatinine
- GFR (eGFR)
- Phosphorus
- Potassium
- Sodium
- Uric Acid

Liver/Gail Bladder Individual Function Tests

- Alkaline phosphatase
- Bilirubin
- BUN
- Cholesterol, total
- Coagulation Panel
- GGT
- LDH Cholesterol
- 5'-Nucleotidase
- Platelet Count
- Pro Time
- Serum Protein
- SGOT (AST)
- SGPT (ALT)
- Total Proteins

Pathogen Serology Tests

- AIDS/HIV
- Antibody tests
- Blood group
- ELISA allergy test
- Lyme disease
- Pregnancy tests
- Rheumatoid factor (RF)
- Rh Factor
- Western blot

Pregnancy Tests

Values will Decrease
- Albumin
- Bcarbonate
- Calcium
- Creatinine
- HgB, HCT
- Phosphorus
- SGOT (AST)
- Sodium

Values will Increase
- Alkaline Phosphatase
- Chloride
- Cholesterol
- Glucose
- LDH
- Sedimentation rate
- White blood cells (WBC)

---

pH Values

Alkalinity
- 7.0 Neutral Water
- 7.0-higher Green drinks, vegetables, lemons, spinach
- 7.1 Saliva
- 7.34 Blood
- 7.45 Mother's breast milk
- 7.8 Bottled water
- 9.0 Sea water
- 10.0 Baking soda

Acidity
- 1.0 Sulfuric acid
- 1.5 Stomach acid
- 2.5 Cola
- 3.2 Diet Cola
- 3.9 Sugar
- 4.0 Caffeine
- 4.6 Green tea
- 4.7 Beer
- 4.9 Meat, animal protein

Thyroid Function Tests

- Free Thyroid Index (FTI)
- T3
- Free T3
- T4
- Free T4
- Thyroid antibody tests
- Thyroid Binding Globulin (TBG)
- Thyroid Globulin
- Thyroid Peroxidase
- Thyroid Stimulating Hormone (TSH)
- Thyroxine, serum

Cancer Serum Tests

- Alpha Fetoprotein (AFP)
- Cancer Antigen CA-125
- Cancer Antigen CA-15-3
- Cancer Antigen CA-19.9
- Carcinoembryonic Antigen (CEA)
- Prostate Specific Antigen (PSA)

MEASUREMENTS

g: grams
g/dL: grams per deciliter
mcg: micrograms
mg/dL: milligrams per decimeter
ng: nanograms
pg: pictograms
L: liter
dL: deciliter (1/10 of a liter= 100 ml)
fl: fraction of one-millionth of a liter
mEq/L: milliequivalents per liter
ml: milliliter (1/1000 of a liter)
mmol/L: millimoles per liter
U: unit
mcmol/L: micromoles per liter
mcU: microunit
IU: international unit
IU/ml: international units per milliliter
mIU/L: milli-international units per liter
mlU/ml: milli-international units per millimeter
u/ML: units per milliliter
Mm: millimeter
cmm: cells per cubic millimeter
mmHg: millimeters of mercury
mm3: cubic millimeters
mEq: milliequivalents
micron: micrometer
mM: millimoles
ng/ml: nanograms per milliliter
PG/ml: one–trillionth of a gram (pictogram)

INDEX

Aafp.org

Alternative News Project

Americanpregnancy.org

Amymyersmd.com

Aruplab.com

Babymed.com

Balch, P.A., Balch James F., *Prescription for Nutritional Healing,* 3rd edition, Penguin Putnam, Inc, NY, 2000

Bcw.edu

Biomedcentral.com

Britannica.com

Buhner, SH, *Herbal Antibiotics,* Storey Publishing, North Adams, MA, 2012

Buhner, SH, *Herbal Antivirals,* Storey Publishing, North Adams, MA, 2013

Buzzle.com

Candidasupport.org

Cdc.gov

Chemcare.com

Connealy, LE, *Blood Tests Results: Your Guide to Understanding the Results,* Sonaraquest.com

Diagnose-me.com

Drhyman.com

Drweil.com

Duke, JA, *The Green Pharmacy*, Rodale Press, Emmeus, PA, 1997

Ehow.com

Emedicine.medscape.com

Firstdescents.org

Gifford, N.L., *Common Blood Tests,* 3rd edition, TBL, Inc, Lake Grove, NY, 1996

Goldberg, B, Diamond, WJ, Cowden, WL, *Cancer,* Future Medicine Publishing, Tiburon, CA, 1997

Grannymedicine.com

Greatist.com/grow/guide-blood-test-results

Healthcaremagic.com

Healthline.com

Healthtap.com

Healthwatchersnews.com

Healyourselfathome.com

Heart.org

Heyman, A. "Testosterone, Cortisol, and Insulin", Townsend Letter #348, July 2012, 50-54

Herbalgram.com

Holistichelp.net

Home-remedies-for-you.com

HSS.edu

Huber, G. "Metabolic Syndrome and Cardiovascular Disease", Townsend Letter #358, May, 2013. 52-60

Igancure.com

Insidetracker.com

Kharrazian, D., Functional Blood Chemistry Analysis, lecture notes, 2005

Kidneycoach.com

Kidney.support.com

Labtestsonline.org

Lifeextension.com

Linus Pauling Institute Research Newsletter

Livestrong.com

Luna, A. How to Make Your Body Alkaline (and Why), Alternative News Project, March 19, 2016, tinyurl.com

Marion, Joseph B, Anti-Aging Manual, Information Pioneers Publishing, South Woodstock, 2003

Mayoclinic.org

Mayomedeicalcolaborative.com

McCarthy, MF. "Manipulating Tumor Acidification as a Cancer Treatment Stategy", Alternative Medicine Review, 15(3), 264-269.

Medhelp.org

Medicinenet.com

Medicine Plus (nim.nih.gov)

Medscape.com

Melamed, PM, Melamed, FM, "Acidity Kills the Pancreas", Townsend Letter, Aug/Sept 2015. 74-80.

Merckmanual.com

Mercola.com

Merriam-Webster.com

Metafilter.com

Modern Essentials, Fourth Edition. Aroma Tools, Orem, UT, 2012

Modern Essentials, Seventh Edition. Aroma Tools, Orem, UT, 2016

Nature-hormones.net

Naturalnews.com

Naturalsociety.com

Naturopathic.org

Newportnaturalhealth.com

Nmslabs.com

Questdiagnostics.com

Rau, T. Biological Medicine, Semmelweis-Institut, Hasseler Steinweg 9, Germany, 2011

Renal.com

Sonaraquest.com

Speedyremedies.com

Tai, PL. "Monthly Miracles", Townsend Letter #358, May, 2013. 109-111

Townsendletter.com

Uptodate.com

Viadro, C. "Sulphate, Sleep, Sunlight and Glyphosate", Nexus, 21(5); 19-24

Watt, SW. "Low Ferritin Epidemic", Nexus, 21(5); 25-28

WebMD.com

Werthmann, K. Sanum Therapy Prescription Book, Semmel-Verlas, Hoga, Germany, 2003

Wikihow.com

Wikipedia.org

Wright, J. The Anticancer Testosterone Metabolite, Townsend Letter #348. July 2012. 55

ABOUT THE AUTHOR

Dr. Daniel T. Wagner is a 1975 graduate of the School of Pharmacy at Duquesne University in Pittsburgh. He received an international MBA in 1993, and attained a Doctorate of Pharmacy degree from Ohio Northern University in 2000.

Dr. Wagner is the recipient of numerous awards and recognitions. Most notably, he was honored as the "Pennsylvania Pharmacist of the Year" in 1996 by the Pennsylvania Pharmacists Association. In 1999, he was recognized by American Druggist Magazine as one of the "Fifty Most Influential Pharmacists in America." In August 2000, *Drug Topics*, a nationally distributed news magazine for pharmacists, named Dr. Dan among their "Pharmacists of the Year 2000." Also in 2000, Dr. Dan was the recipient of the "American Pharmaceutical Association 2000 Merit Award", their highest national award to recognize outstanding service in the field of pharmacy practice.

After 17 years as the owner of an independent community pharmacy, Dan Wagner opened NutriFARMACY in April 1997, a new concept pharmacy specializing in nutrition, wellness and healthcare. In Spring 2016, he sold his natural pharmacy business and still maintains a private practice in holistic and integrative medicine. He incorporates a number of state-of-the-art frequency machines (e.g., ETAscan, REBA, Oligoscan, Quantum Resonance Analyzer, ITOVI) into his health evaluations, coupled with homeopathic and biomedicines from Europe, to evaluate energetic imbalances in patients. He treats patients both in person at via distance.

Dan has done extensive traveling and research on plant medicines in the rain forests of Belize, Peru, Costa Rica, Ecuador, Cuba and western Africa, and has incorporated his knowledge and experience into his natural medicine practice. He is the co-founder and president of The Student Rainforest Fund (SRF) a nonprofit educational organization that enables college students (studying the health professions) to visit the rainforests of Central and South America. SRF is now in its twentieth year. Dr. Dan is also president of The World Health Vision, an NGO that travels to Third World countries in Africa and South American doing humanitarian programs to promote health and well being.

**Dr. Dan can be reached at Askdrdanwagner@gmail.com.
Visit his blog at Askdrdanwagner.info.**

Made in the USA
Coppell, TX
08 August 2021